AF228945

WHAT ARE PSYCHOTIC DISORDERS?

by Jennifer Phillips

BrightPoint Press

San Diego, CA

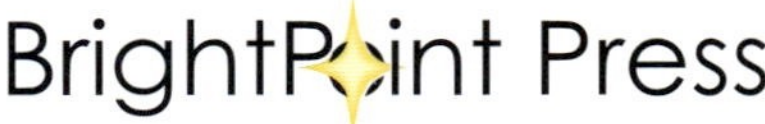

Content Consultant: David Dodell-Feder, PhD, Assistant Professor of Psychology and Neuroscience, University of Rochester

LIBRARY OF CONGRESS CATALOGING-IN-PUBLICATION DATA

Names: Phillips, Jennifer, 1962- author.
Title: What are psychotic disorders? / by Jennifer Phillips.
Description: San Diego, CA : BrightPoint Press, [2023] | Series:
   Understanding disorders | Includes bibliographical references and index.
   | Audience: Grades 10-12
Identifiers: LCCN 2022003974 (print) | LCCN 2022003975 (eBook) |
ISBN 9781678204525 (hardcover) | ISBN 9781678204532 (eBook)
Subjects: LCSH: Psychoses--Juvenile literature. | Psychoses--Treatment--Juvenile literature.
Classification: LCC RC512 .P45 2023 (print) | LCC RC512 (eBook) | DDC
   616.89--dc23/eng/20220203
LC record available at https://lccn.loc.gov/2022003974
LC eBook record available at https://lccn.loc.gov/2022003975

CONTENTS

AT A GLANCE

- Psychotic disorders are rare mental health conditions. They affect less than 1 percent of US adults.

- Psychosis is the main symptom of psychotic disorders. It can cause false beliefs called delusions. It can also cause someone to see or hear something that isn't there.

- There are many types of psychotic disorders. Schizophrenia is the most common.

- People with schizophrenia may experience delusions and hallucinations. They may have disorganized speech. They may struggle to take care of themselves.

- Other psychotic disorders include schizophreniform disorder and schizoaffective disorder. Brief psychotic disorder and delusional disorder are some examples.

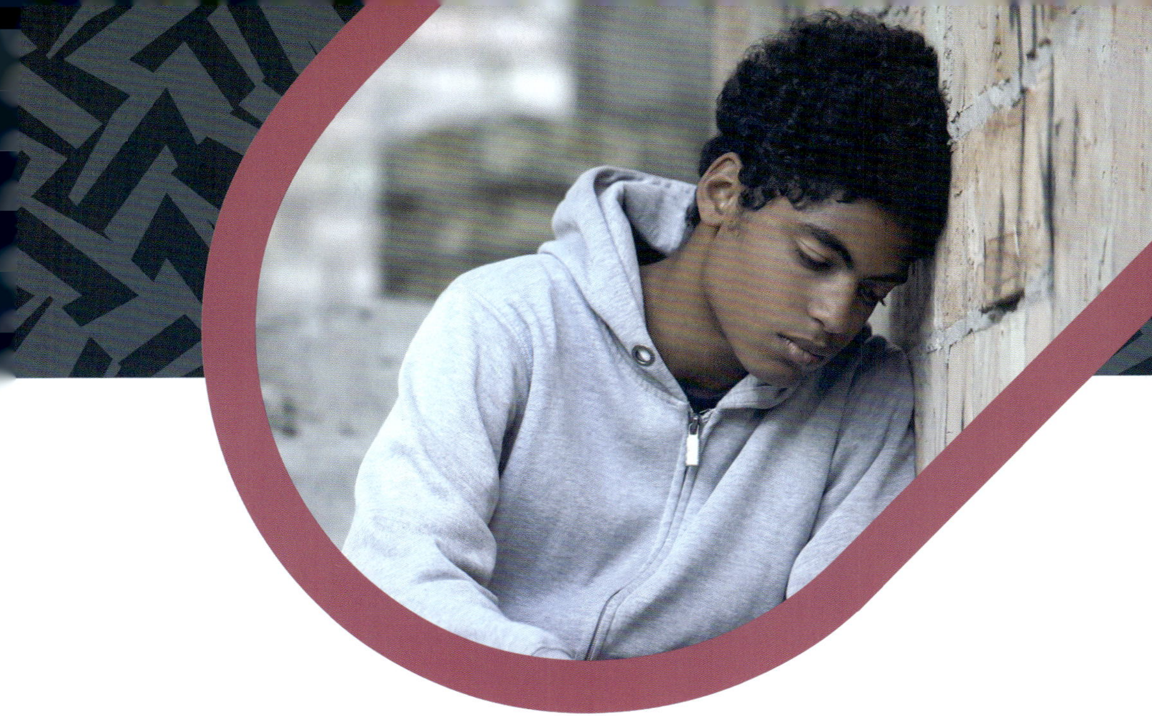

- Many factors are linked to psychotic disorders. Family history and brain abnormalities can increase the risk of developing a psychotic disorder.

- Antipsychotic drugs are commonly used to treat psychotic disorders. These drugs help change levels of brain chemicals.

- Psychotherapy is another form of treatment for psychotic disorders. Therapists work with patients to help them cope with symptoms and reduce stress.

- Scientists research ways to treat specific symptoms of psychotic disorders.

LIVING WITH SCHIZOPHRENIA

Cecilia McGough was a successful science student. She codiscovered a star. She participated in the International Space Olympics. But things changed during her freshman year of college. "My life had become a waking nightmare," she said in a 2017 TEDx Talk.[1] She talked about her experience with mental illness.

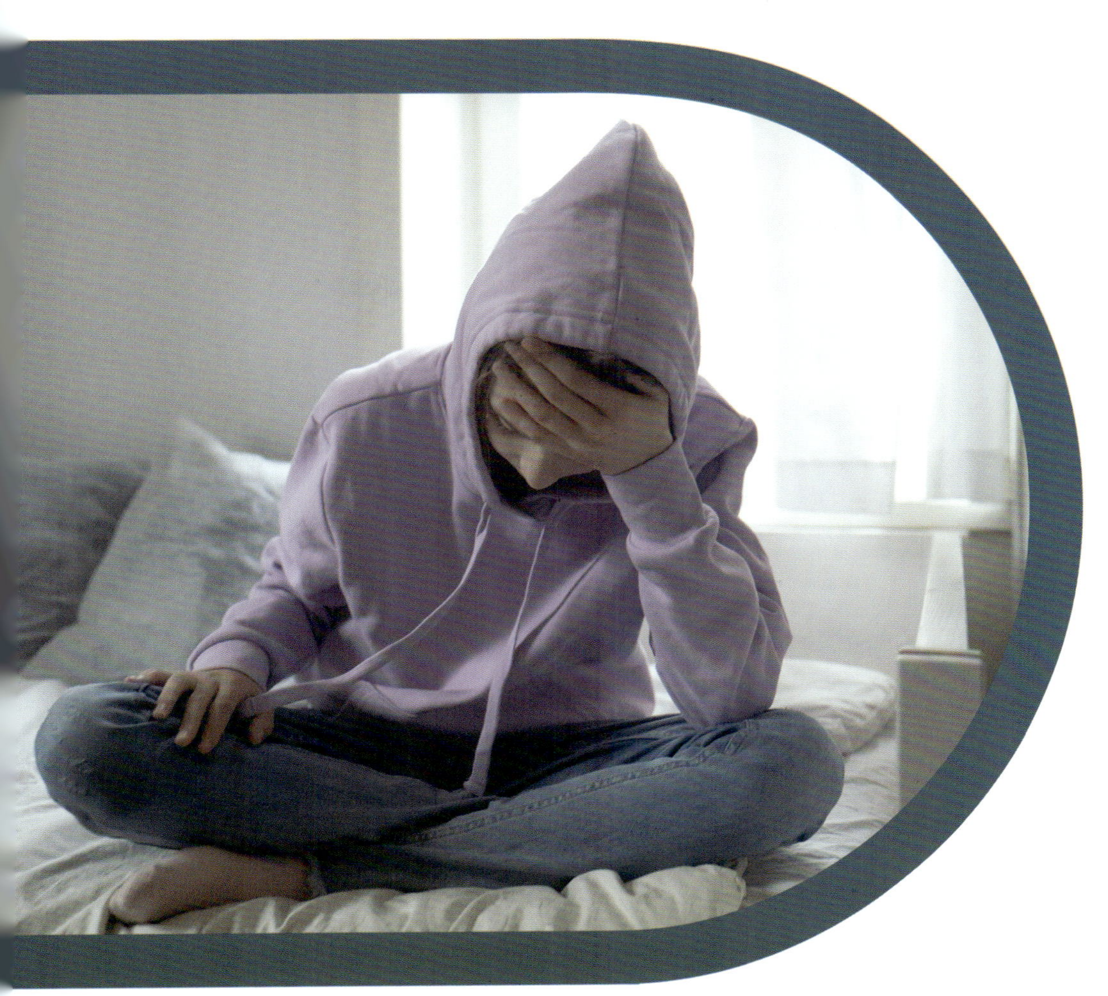

Spending less time with others can be a warning sign of schizophrenia.

Cecilia saw things that were not real. She first saw shadowy figures when she was a young girl. She heard whispers as a teen. She struggled with scattered thoughts.

Her **hallucinations** became worse. She saw an evil clown. She saw a girl who stabbed her in the face with a knife.

Cecilia tried to keep these symptoms a secret. Eventually they became unbearable. She couldn't concentrate in school. She was filled with fear and doubt. Cecilia needed special care. She was **diagnosed** with schizophrenia. "Getting medical help was the best decision that I have ever made," Cecilia shared.[2]

ABOUT PSYCHOTIC DISORDERS

Psychotic disorders are mental health conditions. They affect people's thoughts.

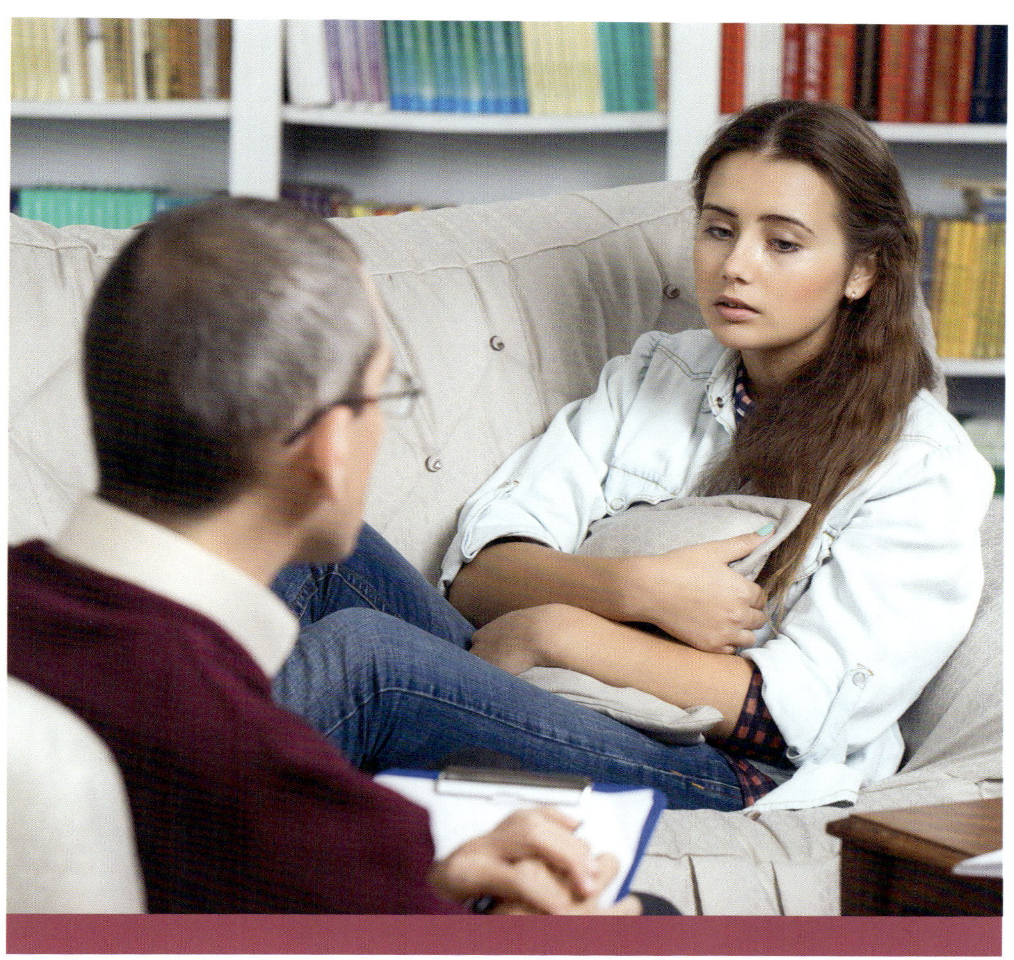

Seeking treatment for psychotic disorders has helped many people ease their symptoms.

They can cause people to see and hear things that are not real. Schizophrenia is one type of psychotic disorder. There are many others. Psychosis is the main

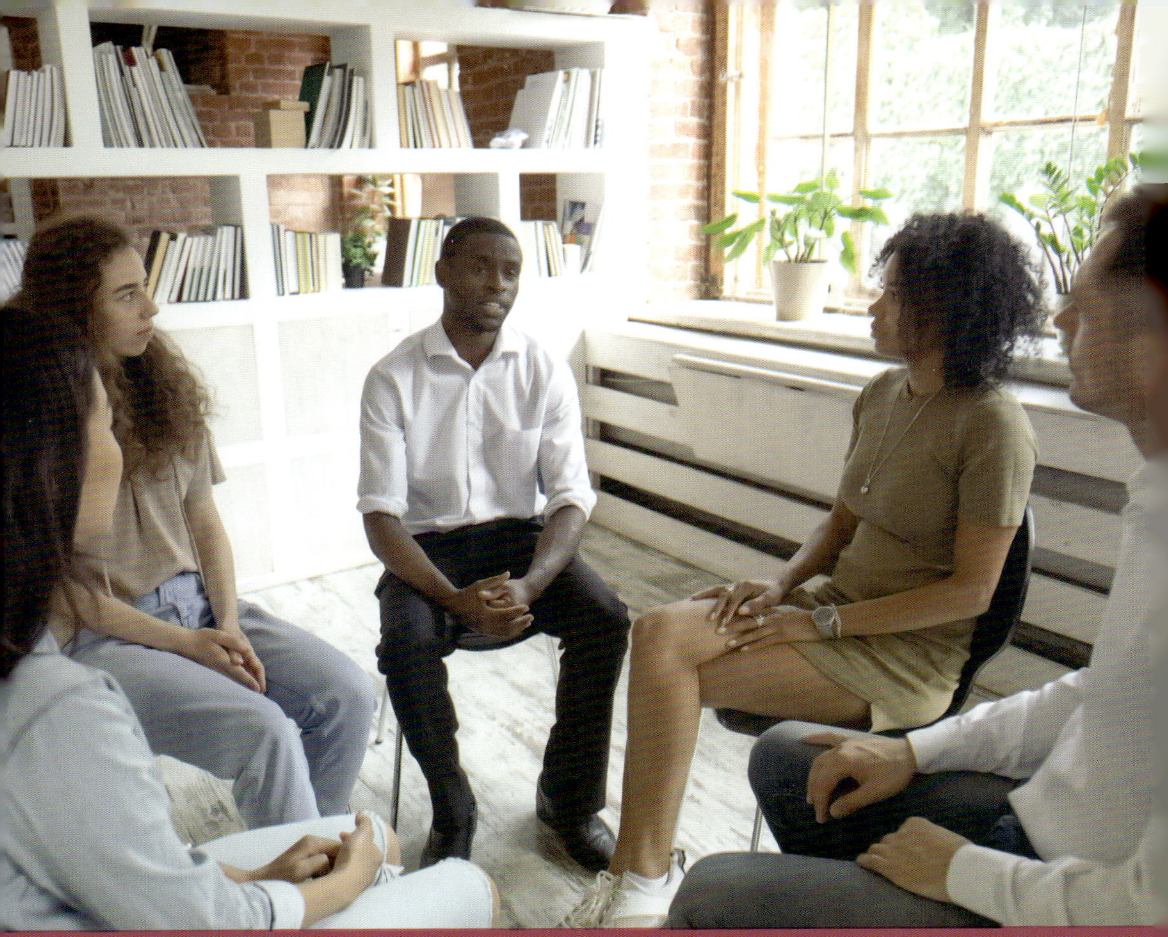

symptom of these disorders. This is when

someone loses touch with reality.

Psychotic disorders are rare. Less than

1 percent of US adults have a psychotic

disorder. These disorders can have serious

impacts if left untreated. It is critical to share symptoms with a doctor.

Social support is also important. People may feel ashamed of their symptoms. They may feel as if nobody understands them. "In college, I tried to go to different mental health clubs. But no one was really talking about hallucinations," Cecilia said.[3] She launched Students with Psychosis. This organization supports college students. It helps them understand psychosis. Cecilia shares her story. She encourages others who live with a psychotic disorder.

CHAPTER ONE

THE HISTORY OF PSYCHOTIC DISORDERS

Psychotic disorders may have been described as early as 3,000 years ago. Chinese writings from that time described people experiencing confusion. They also had hallucinations.

Hippocrates was an ancient Greek doctor. He introduced new ideas about

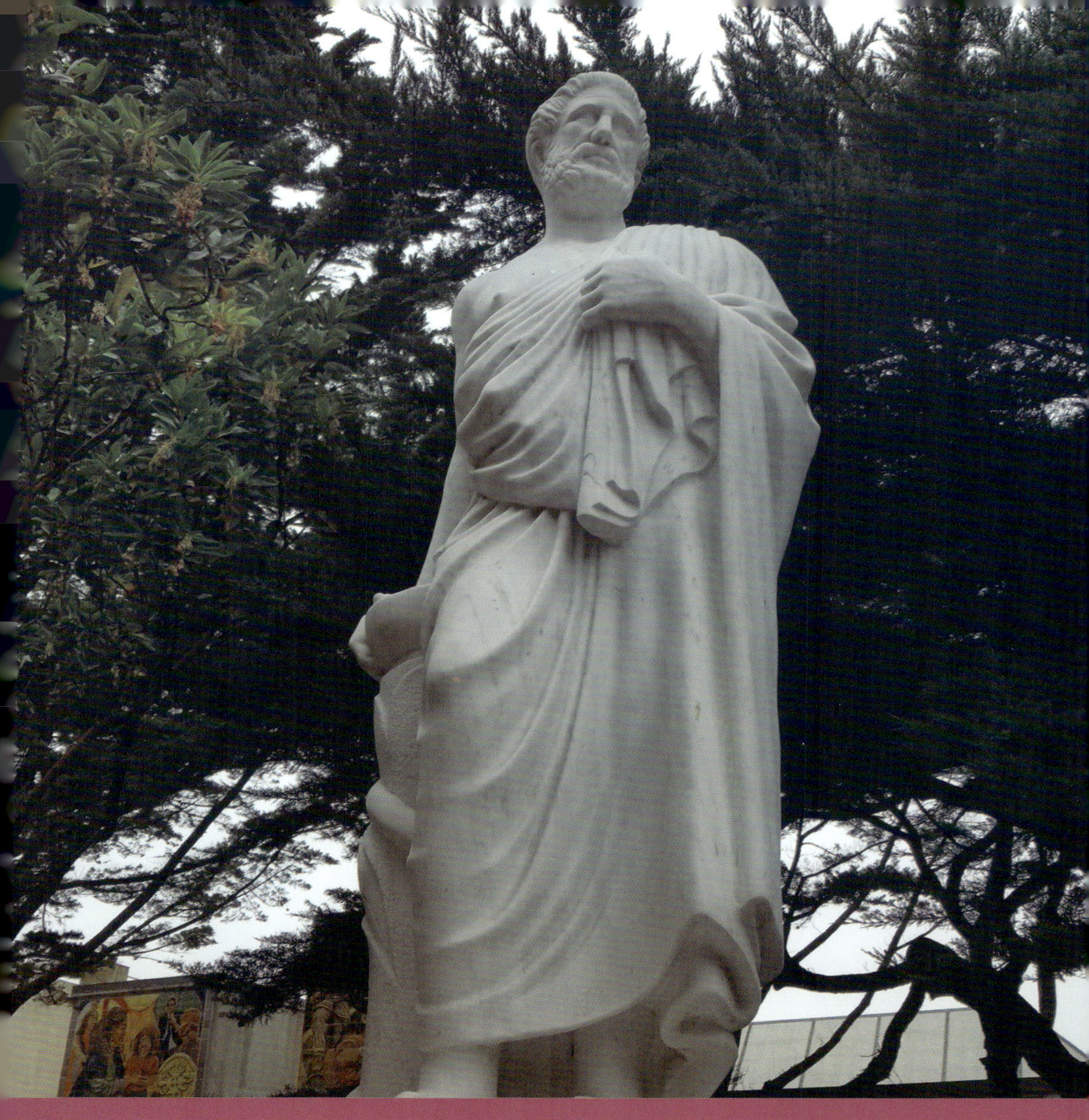

Hippocrates played a large role in ancient mental health research.

mental illness. He thought the balance of

bodily fluids affected health. He believed

that changes in blood levels could affect a person's happiness. Hippocrates also created the first classifications for mental health disorders. He described a mental disorder he called paranoia. This is a feeling of intense distrust. It can describe some symptoms of schizophrenia today.

MODERN UNDERSTANDING OF PSYCHOTIC DISORDERS

Doctors first used the term *psychosis* in 1845. It described a variety of symptoms. These symptoms included confusion and scattered thoughts. They also included hallucinations. Dr. Emil Kraepelin

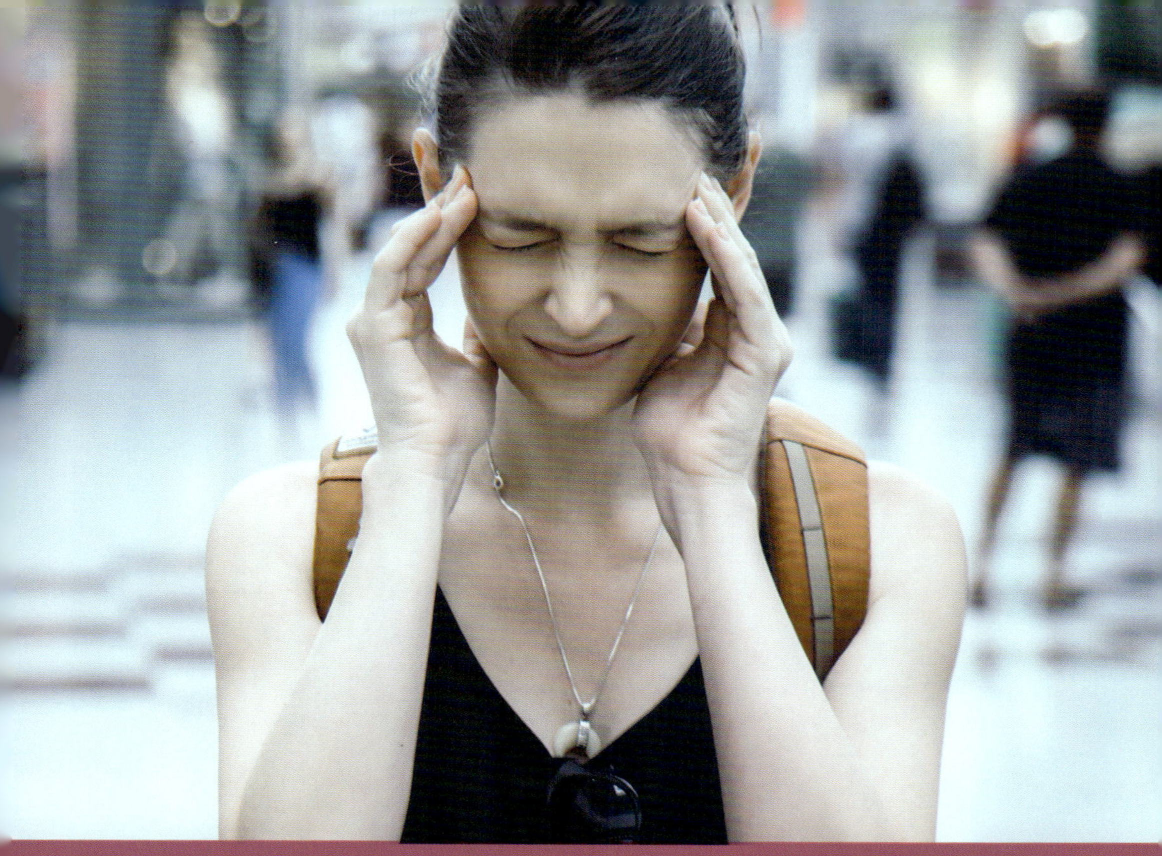

Hearing voices is a common hallucination.

identified two disorders that could cause

psychosis. This symptom lasted for a

short time in some of his patients. It was

more permanent in others. He called the

long-lasting form "dementia praecox." Today

the disorder is known as schizophrenia.

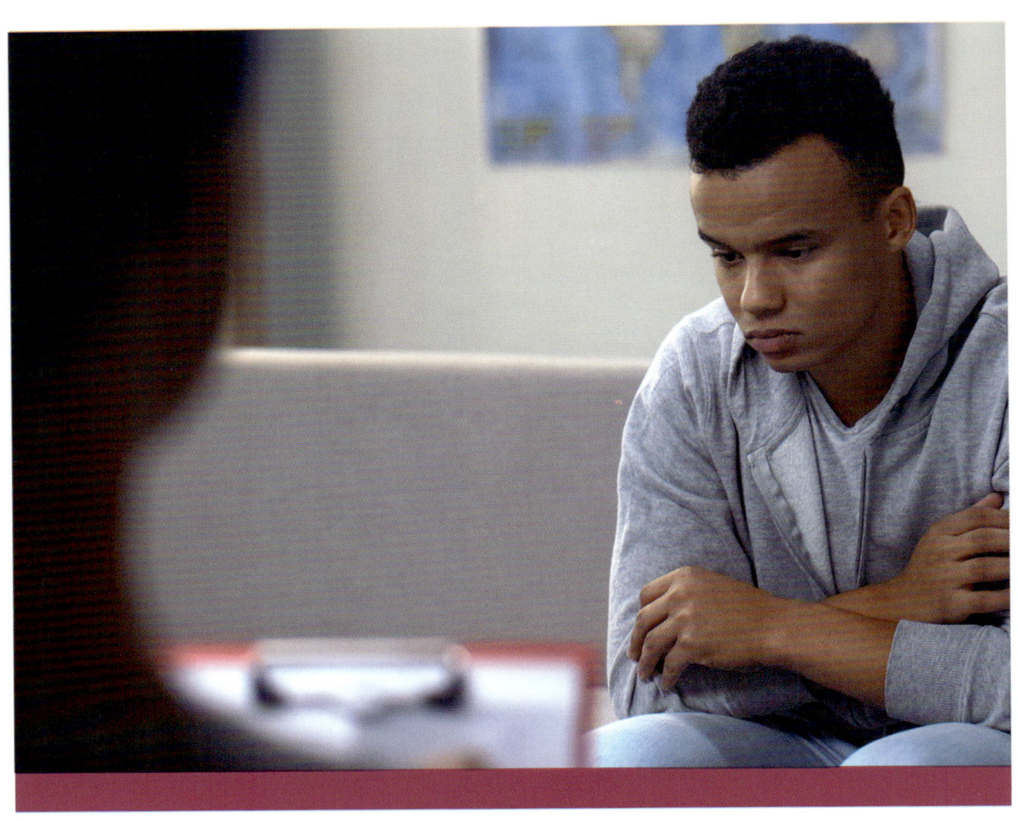

Schizophrenia affects everyone differently.

Eugen Bleuler was a psychiatrist. He was the first person to use the term *schizophrenia*. He created it in 1911. The word has Greek roots. *Schizo* means "split." *Phrene* means "mind." This described the scattered thoughts of his patients.

Researchers continued to learn more about psychotic disorders. The American Psychiatric Association (APA) published a book in 1952. It was the *Diagnostic and Statistical Manual of Mental Disorders* (*DSM*). Doctors use this book to diagnose mental health disorders. It includes information on psychotic disorders.

Scientists research mental health. They learn more about mental health disorders. The APA makes updates to the *DSM*. These updates give doctors accurate information. The *DSM-5* is the most recent version as of 2022.

Early versions of the *DSM* listed different types of schizophrenia. But the descriptions of these types were not clear. They didn't help doctors make treatment decisions. The *DSM-5* describes a **spectrum** of schizophrenia disorders. This change shows that there are many symptoms of schizophrenia. These symptoms can range from mild to severe.

EARLY TREATMENTS

Early Greek doctors believed physical health influenced mental health. They suggested exercise to treat mental health. They also recommended a proper diet. Hippocrates

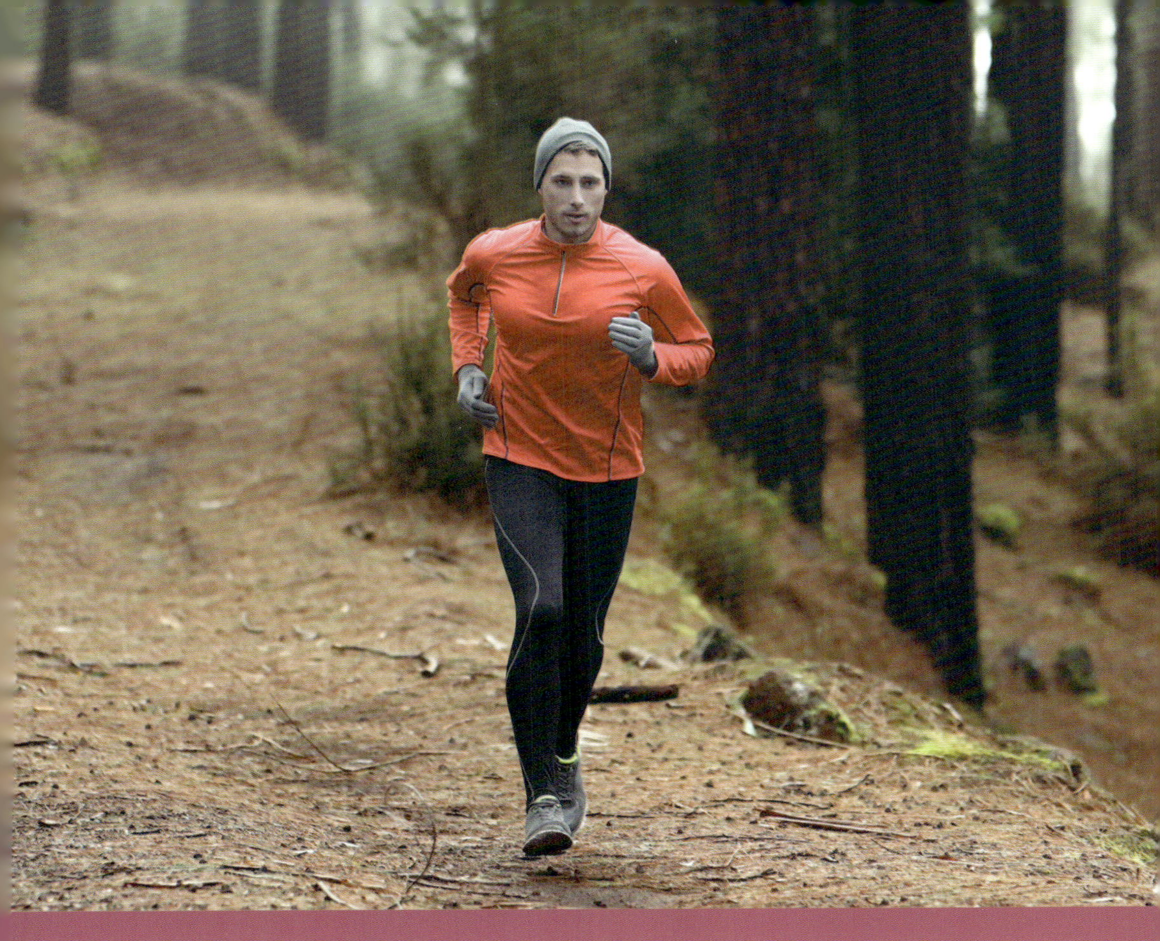

believed that levels of bodily fluids caused

illness. His treatments focused on the

balance of these fluids.

During the Middle Ages, people with

psychotic disorders were treated harshly.

Some people believed demons caused the symptoms. They thought people with mental illnesses were witches. They held people with psychosis in dungeons during this period.

CHANGES IN TREATMENT

Many people with psychotic disorders were held in **asylums** in the 1800s. They were treated like prisoners. Asylum workers kept patients in chains. Many people did not think mental illnesses could be treated.

Dorothea Dix visited asylums in the mid-1800s. She spoke out against the conditions. She wrote to lawmakers,

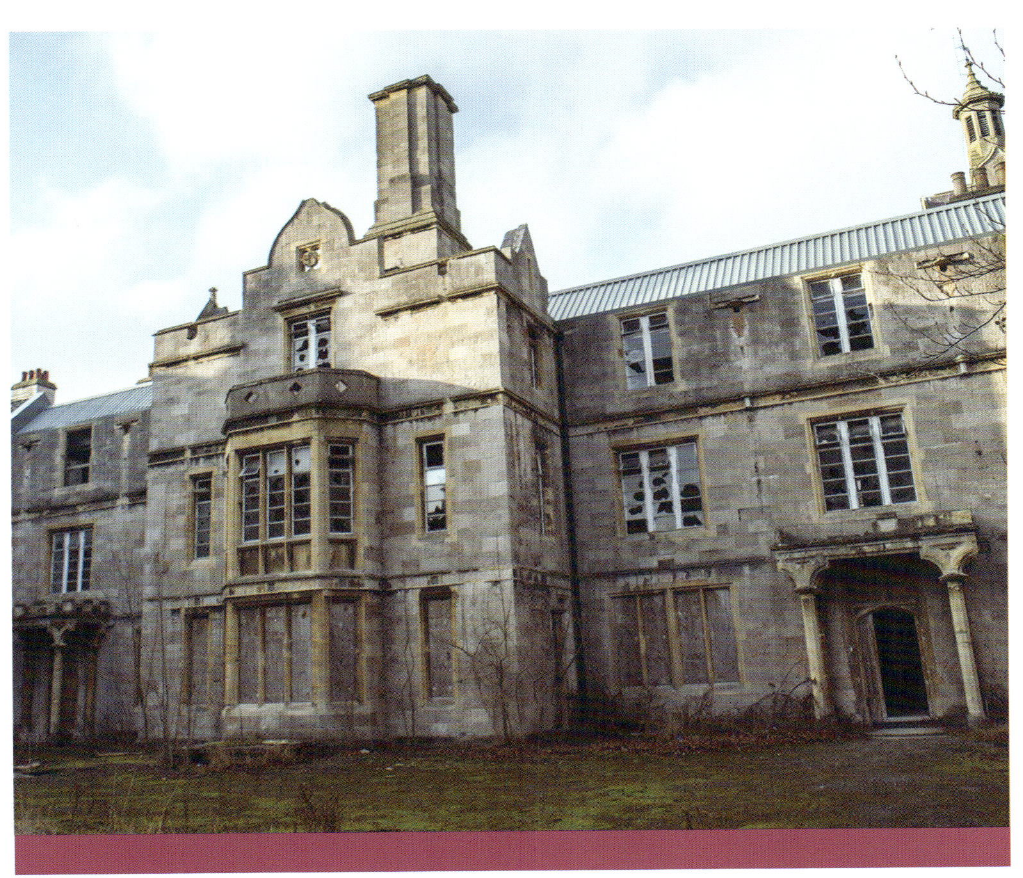

Asylum workers in the 1800s used cruel treatments on their patients.

"I . . . call your attention to the [people] in cages. . . . Chained, naked, beaten with rods, and lashed into obedience!"[4] Dix changed the way mental illness was treated in the United States. More than thirty

mental hospitals were established due to
Dix's efforts.

Doctors used an early form of
electroconvulsive therapy (ECT) to treat
patients. They applied electric shocks to
patients' brains. ECT relieved psychosis. But
some doctors used ECT to punish patients.

A NATIONAL TURNING POINT

President Harry Truman signed the National
Mental Health Act on July 3, 1946. The act
improved mental health care. Mental health
professionals received more training. The act
provided money to mental health clinics. It
also created the National Institute of Mental
Health (NIMH). The NIMH researches mental
health disorders.

Research has improved ECT. This treatment is still used today.

Some early treatments were cruel. Doctors performed surgeries called lobotomies. They cut connections in the front of the brain. This area of the brain influences personality. Lobotomies sometimes got rid of psychosis. But they also had severe side effects. Patients experienced personality changes. Some became very sick. Others died because of the surgery.

Doctors began to use a drug called chlorpromazine (CPZ) in 1952. It was

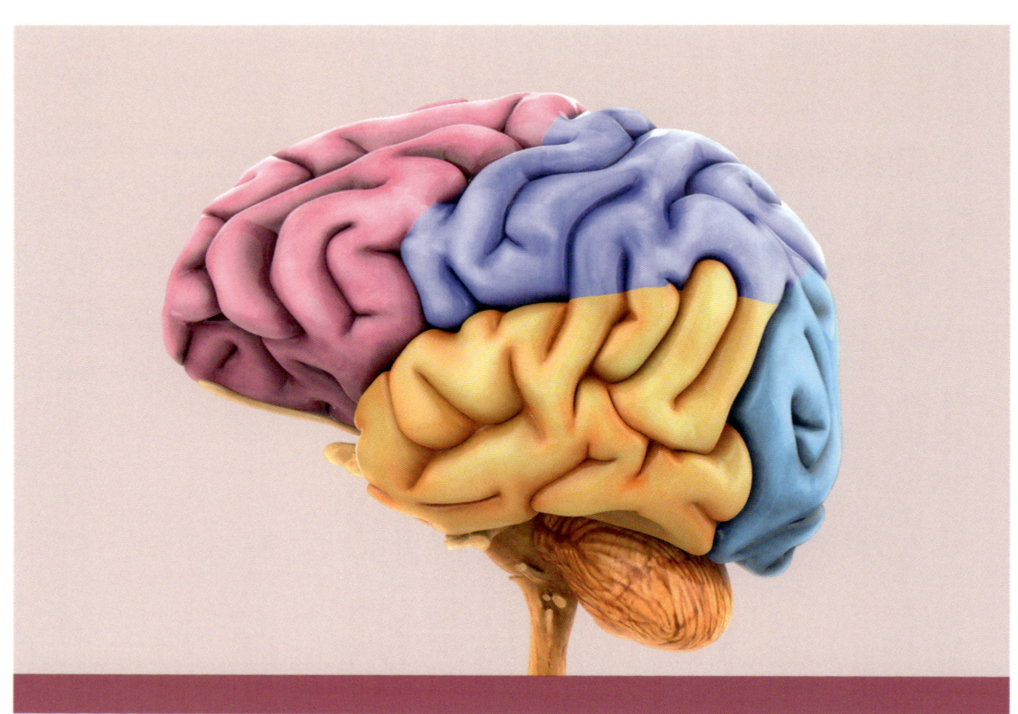

The frontal lobe of the brain (pink) is responsible for functions such as speech, reasoning, and concentration.

the first drug used to treat psychosis.

CPZ proved to be very effective. It is still used to treat psychotic disorders today.

Medication allowed people with psychotic disorders to live stable lives. They no longer needed constant care in mental hospitals. Many began seeking treatment in community programs instead. People began to speak out against mental hospitals. They called attention to cruel treatment. They fought for the right to refuse hospital stays.

THE FIRST ANTIPSYCHOTIC

CPZ was not created to treat psychosis. A French army surgeon started using CPZ to prevent problems during surgery. He noticed it calmed anxious patients. He shared his findings. Doctors used CPZ to treat mania three years later. They also tested it on patients experiencing psychosis. They found CPZ to be extremely effective. But side effects from CPZ can be severe.

The US Supreme Court made a historic ruling in 1975. People with mental illness could not be put in hospitals against their will. They could be forced into a hospital only if they were a danger to themselves or others. Associate Justice Potter Stewart spoke of the decision. He did not support forced hospital stays. Stewart believed it was unjust to "fence in the harmless [people with mental illnesses]." [5]

Scientists continue to learn more about treatments for psychotic disorders. They want to be able to detect the early stages of psychosis. Studies suggest that early

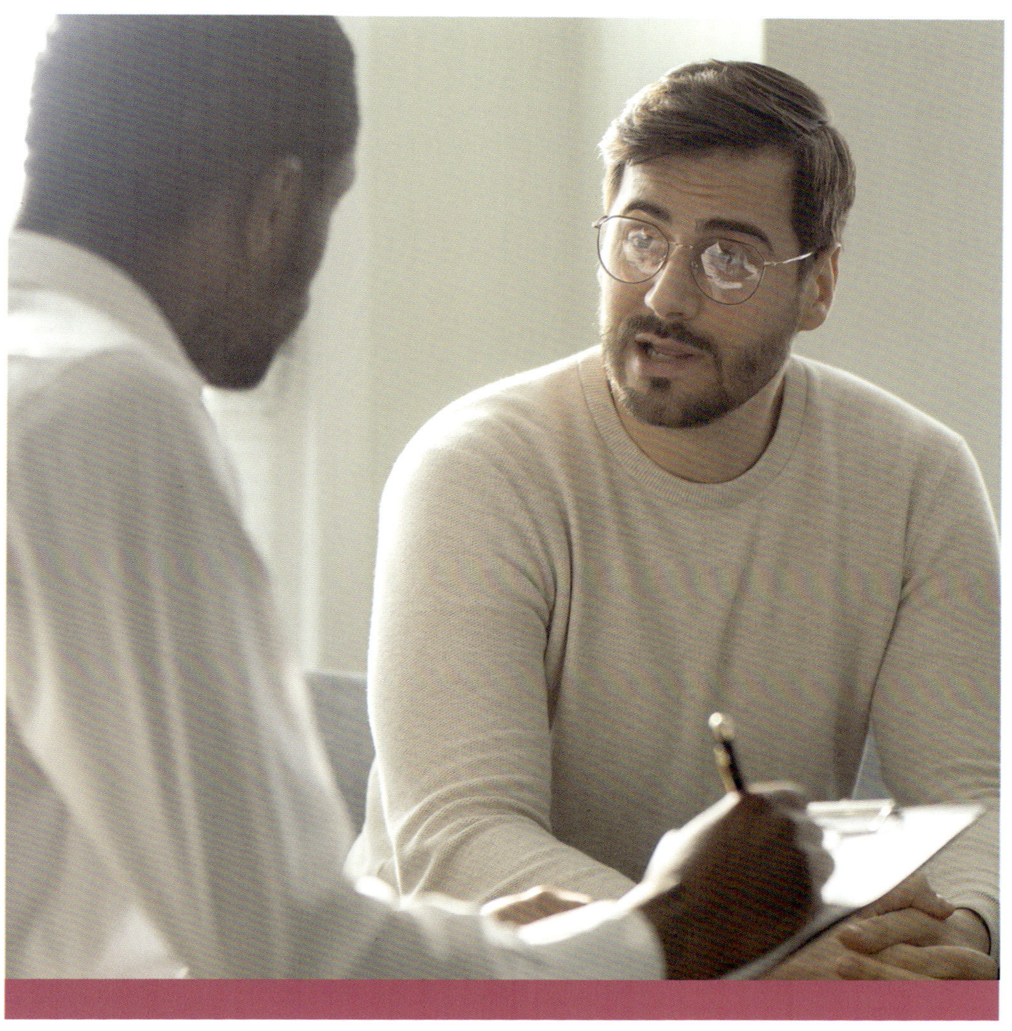

Early treatment of a psychotic disorder can help someone manage symptoms effectively.

detection and treatment improve chances

of recovery.

CHAPTER TWO

NOTABLE PSYCHOTIC DISORDERS

Psychosis is a break from reality. It is the main symptom of psychotic disorders. It causes confusion. Psychosis makes it difficult to know what is real.

Approximately 100,000 US teens and young adults report a first psychotic **episode** each year. Someone who

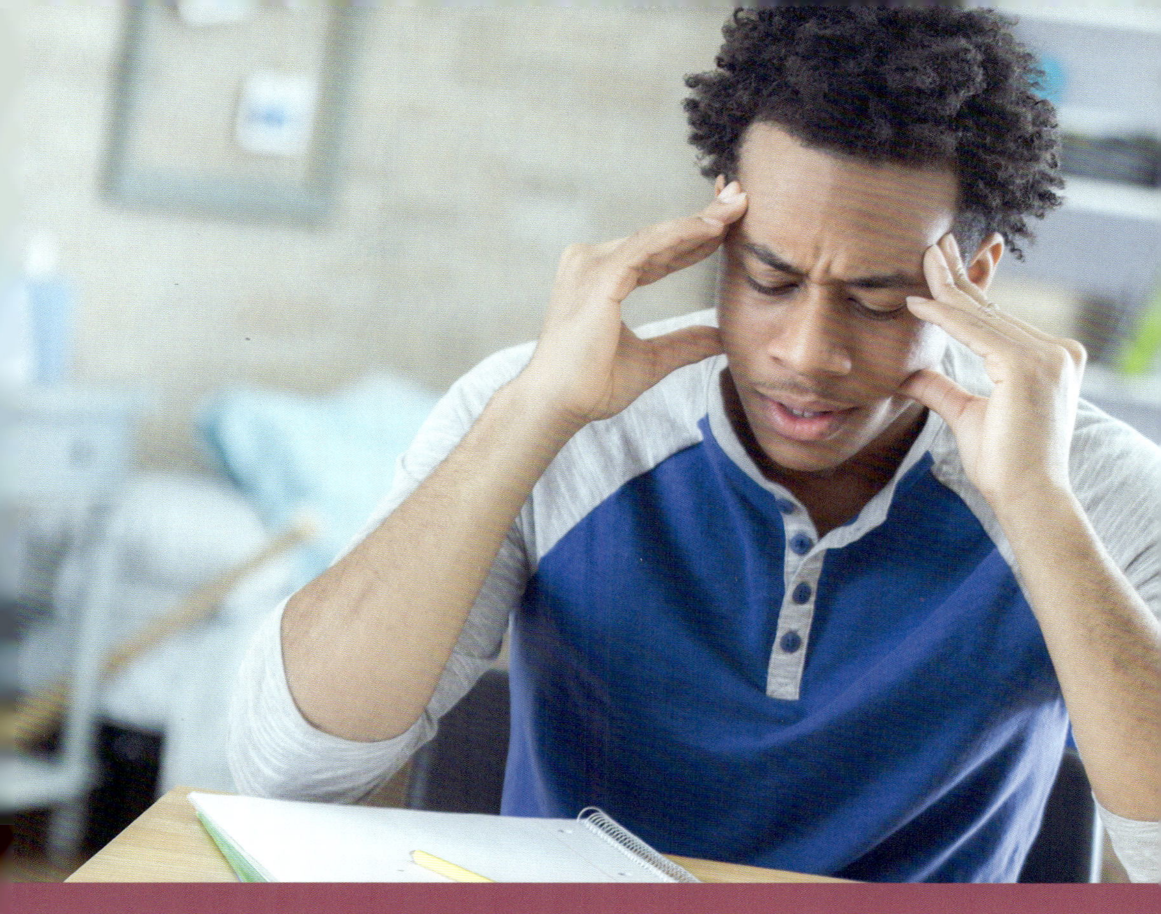

Psychotic disorders can be very disorienting, which can make it difficult to focus.

experiences psychosis may later be

diagnosed with a psychotic disorder.

But other conditions can cause

psychosis. Some people with bipolar

disorder experience psychosis. Health

conditions such as brain tumors can also cause psychosis.

SCHIZOPHRENIA

Schizophrenia is the most common psychotic disorder. But less than 1 percent of the US population has schizophrenia. It tends to be diagnosed in men when they are teens or young adults. Women

EARLY WARNING SIGNS

Psychosis typically occurs gradually. There are warning signs. Someone showing early signs of psychosis may withdraw from others. He may suddenly perform worse at school. He may have a hard time concentrating. It is important to seek medical help if these signs occur.

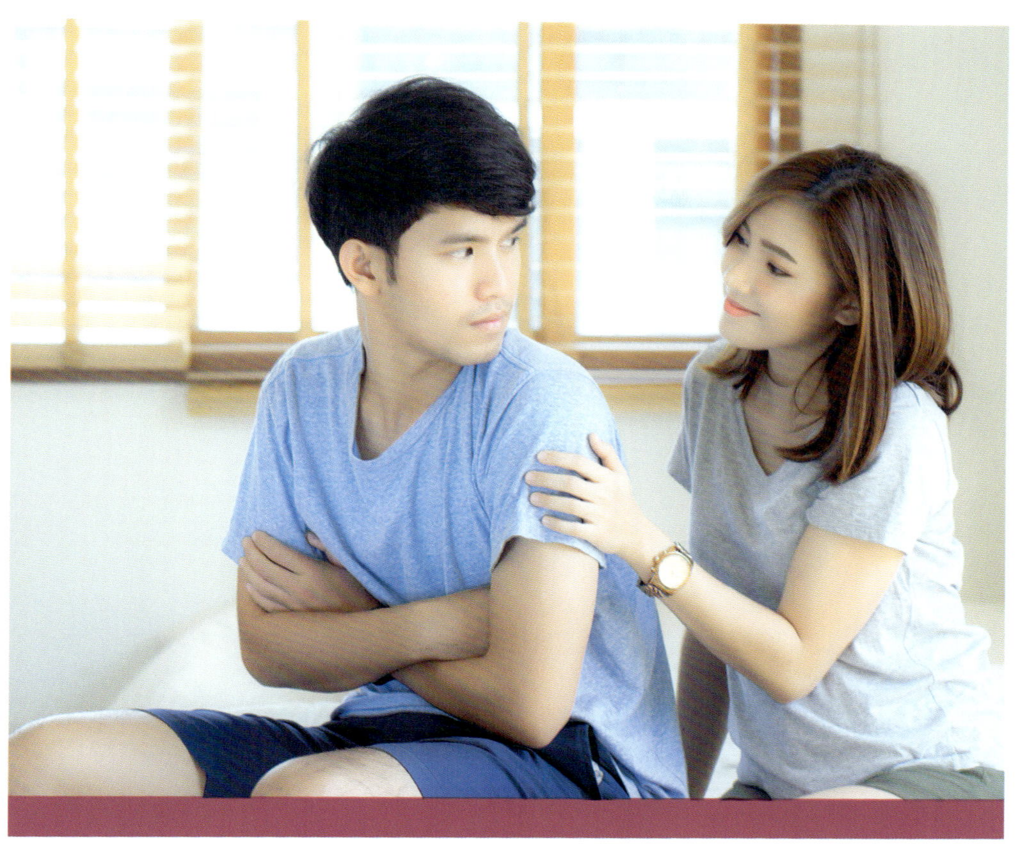

Someone with schizophrenia may be paranoid. He may become distrustful toward people he is close to.

are usually diagnosed in their twenties

or thirties. Psychosis may occur more

rapidly in men. Their symptoms may also

last longer.

There is a wide range of symptoms in schizophrenia. Symptoms range from mild to severe. There are five main symptoms of this disorder.

People with schizophrenia may have delusions. These are untrue beliefs. Delusions make daily life difficult. For example, someone may believe she is under attack. She may think her friends want to hurt her. She does not have evidence for these feelings. But the delusion affects her behavior. She may avoid her friends. There are other common delusions. Some people believe they have special powers.

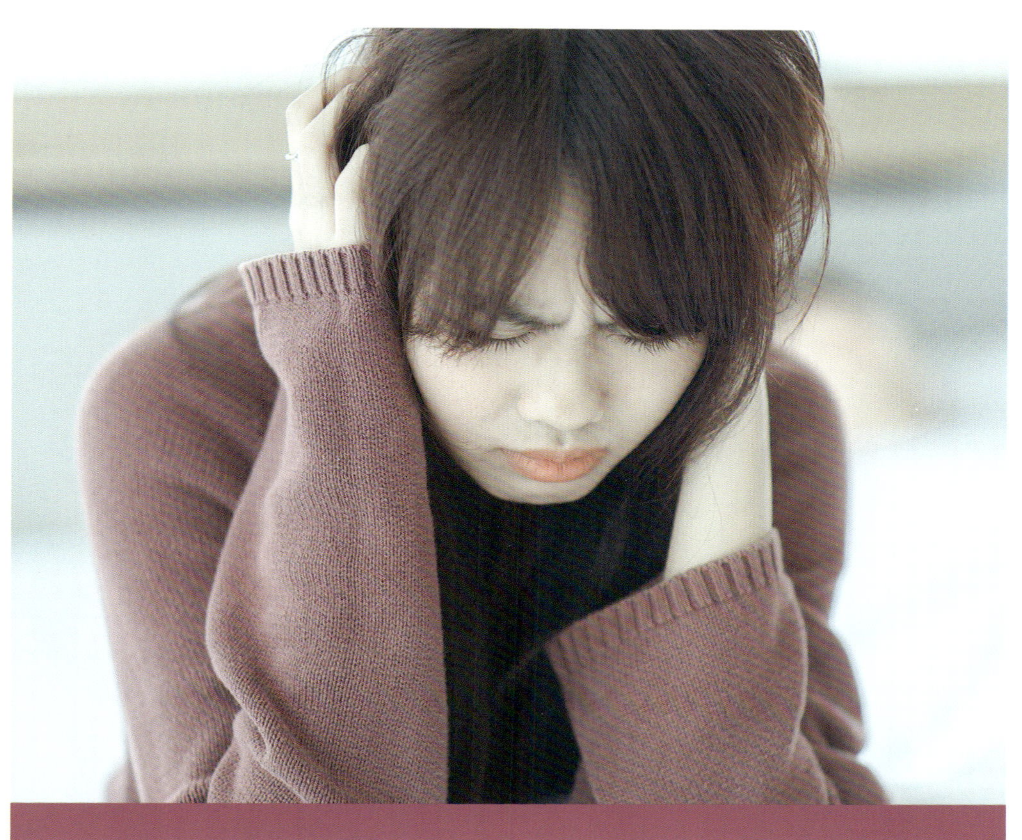

Hallucinations often feel very real to people with a psychotic disorder.

Hallucinations are another symptom. Hearing voices is common. Voices may sound like they come from another person. Or they may sound like they are in a person's mind. Hallucinations can affect other senses. People may see or smell things that aren't there. Touch and taste can also be affected. Some people are able to tell that these experiences are not real. But hallucinations can still be overwhelming.

Someone with schizophrenia may have disorganized speech. He may have a hard time communicating. He may fail to answer questions. Words may not be organized into sentences.

Schizophrenia can also cause disorganized behavior. This behavior includes acting childishly. Someone may get angry easily. She may stay in a

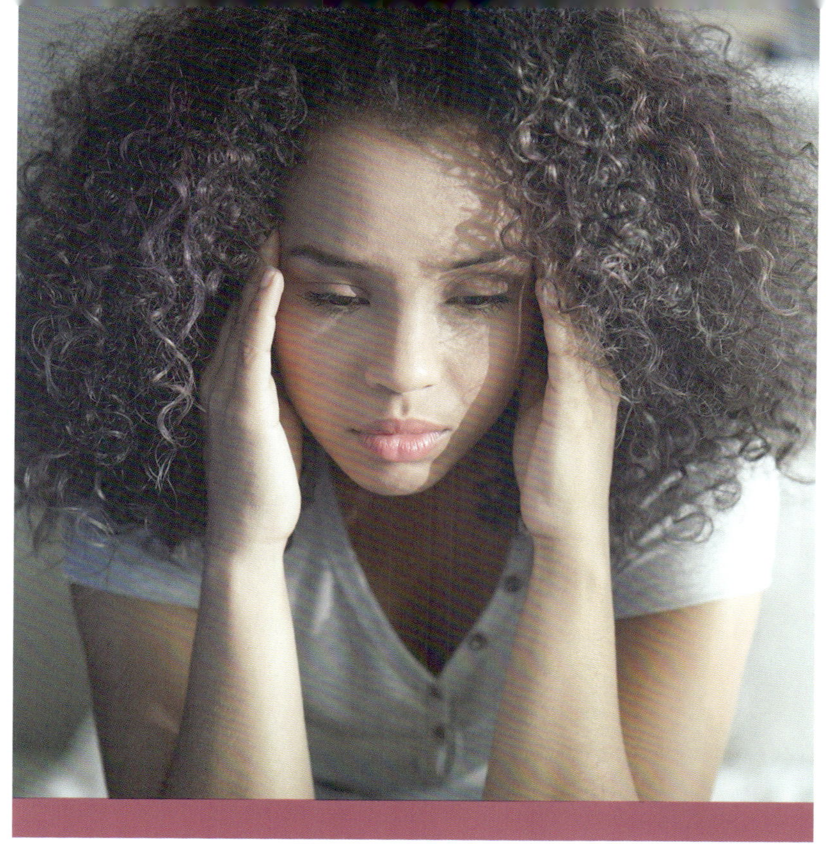

Symptoms of schizophrenia can sometimes be difficult to detect.

rigid position for hours. She may make

unnecessary movements.

The lack of some behaviors can be

a sign of schizophrenia. For example,

someone may have a hard time taking care

of himself. He may not bathe. He may show

little emotion. These are called negative symptoms. They can be difficult to treat.

Someone with schizophrenia must show at least two of these symptoms. These symptoms are severe for at least a month. They may last for a shorter amount of time if the person is taking medication. Signs of schizophrenia must last for six months for a diagnosis. Symptoms are milder during this period. They may be more difficult to notice.

OTHER PSYCHOTIC DISORDERS

Schizophrenia is one type of psychotic disorder. There are others. Many are similar to schizophrenia.

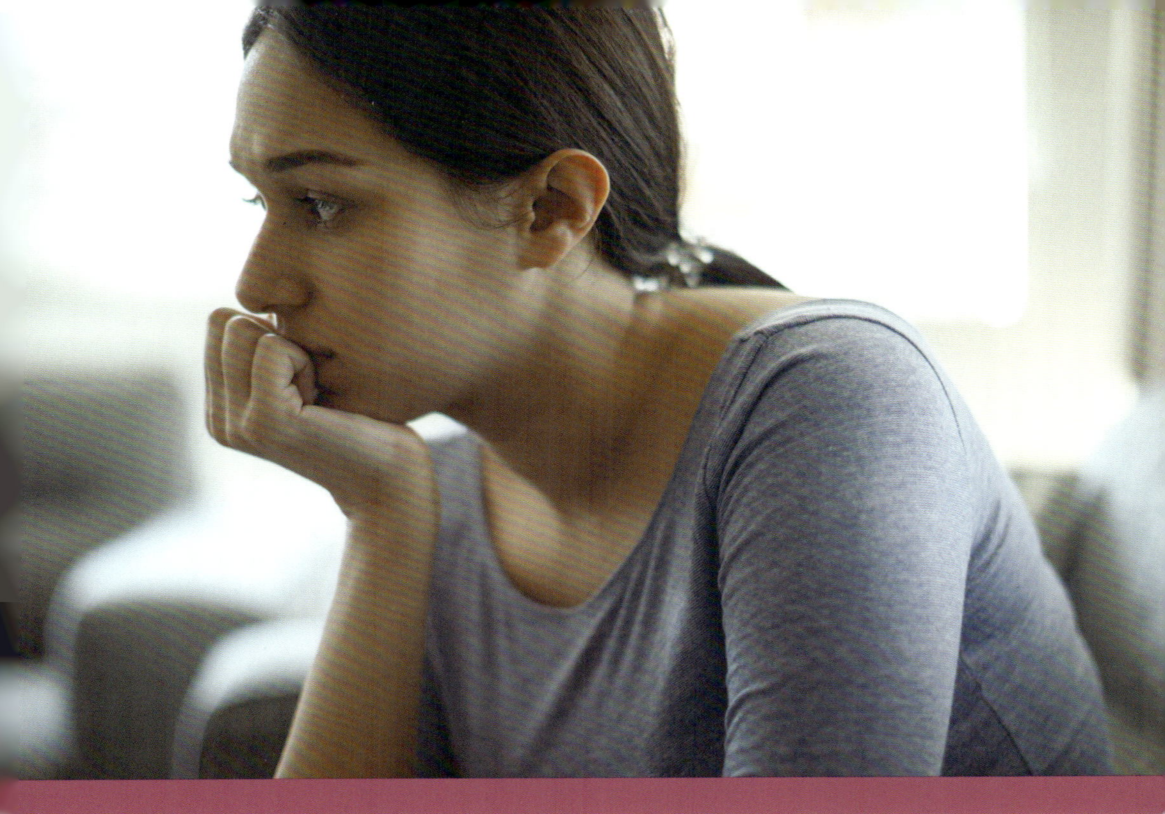

A psychotic disorder can cause severe distress.

Symptoms of schizophreniform disorder are the same as schizophrenia symptoms. But the symptoms last fewer than six months. This is a shorter time than schizophrenia symptoms. About two-thirds of the people with schizophreniform disorder later develop schizophrenia.

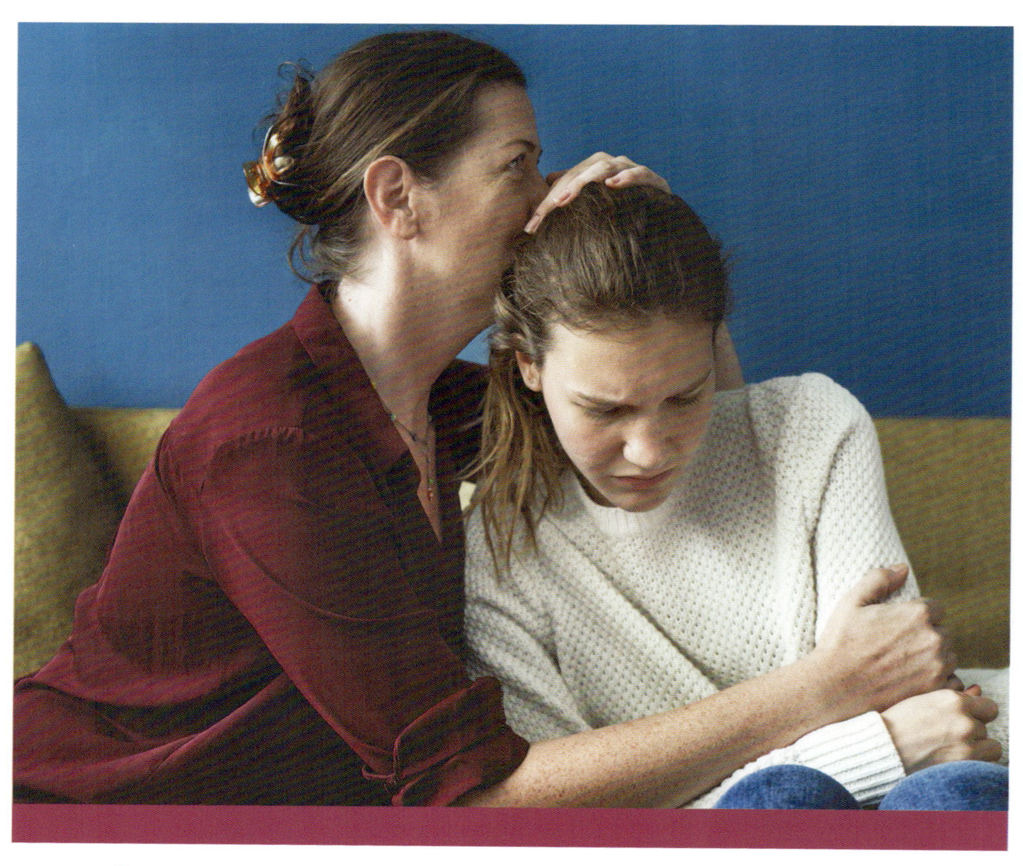

Someone who experiences psychosis may later be diagnosed with schizophrenia.

Schizoaffective disorder is another psychotic disorder. People with this disorder show psychosis. They also show symptoms of a mood disorder. They may be depressed. They may experience mania.

They could have racing thoughts. They may have high energy.

Some people have brief psychotic disorder. Symptoms last for a short period of time. People may recover in less than a month. This disorder is usually caused by extreme stress. The sudden loss of a family member could be a factor.

Delusional disorder is a rare disorder. People with this disorder experience only delusions. They do not show other symptoms. They may think they are being followed. They may become distrustful of others.

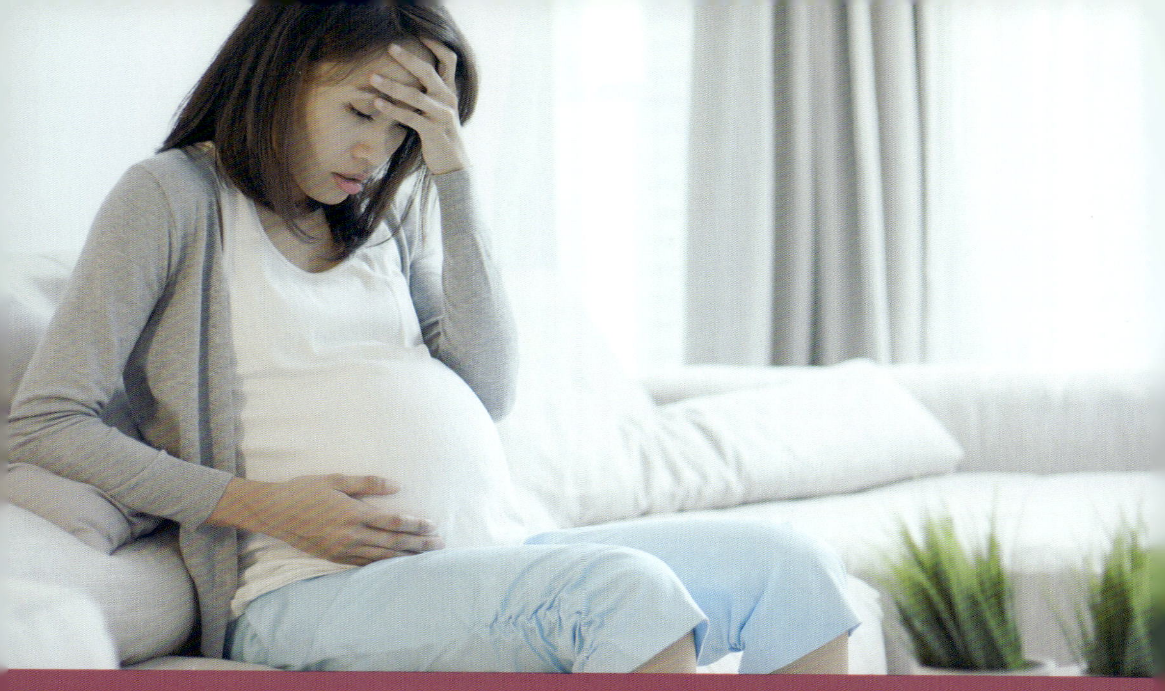

Genetics and issues during pregnancy can play a role in psychotic disorders.

CAUSES OF PSYCHOTIC DISORDERS

Many factors can cause psychotic disorders. Family history is one factor. A parent with schizophrenia is at risk of having a child with the disorder. Scientists have studied the disorder in identical twins. When one twin has the disorder, the other twin is likely to have the disorder too. A person has around a 40 percent chance of developing the disorder if his or her identical twin has it.

Certain illnesses during pregnancy can increase the risk. The child may be more likely to develop a psychotic disorder. Early births increase the risk. Not getting enough oxygen as a fetus is another risk factor.

Schizophrenia is linked to changes in the levels of brain chemicals. A brain chemical called dopamine may be involved. Glutamate and serotonin may also play a role. These brain chemicals may be linked to hallucinations. Dr. Robert

Freedman is a psychiatrist. He talked about how schizophrenia affects the brain. He said, "The brain of someone who has schizophrenia is . . . bombarded with sounds and sights and smells that normally most of us are able to screen out." [6]

External factors play a role in psychotic disorders. Extreme stress can cause psychosis. The loss of a job can be a factor.

SUBSTANCE USE AND PSYCHOSIS

Drug abuse cannot cause schizophrenia. But it can cause psychosis. Drug abuse can lead to addiction and other problems. Drugs can be especially dangerous for people with psychotic disorders. They are more likely to cause psychosis in these people.

The combination of stress and family history can lead to psychotic disorders. Both factors are necessary to develop these disorders.

Psychotic disorders can have a severe impact on life. But scientists are researching the causes of psychotic disorders. Understanding the causes helps inform treatment. Many people with psychotic disorders are able to live happy lives with treatment.

CHAPTER THREE

PSYCHOTIC DISORDERS AND EVERYDAY LIFE

Psychotic disorders can make everyday life difficult. School and work can be challenging. Symptoms may be hard to handle. People with psychotic disorders may also face **stigma**. This can create more challenges. Relationships may suffer. Stigma may cause people

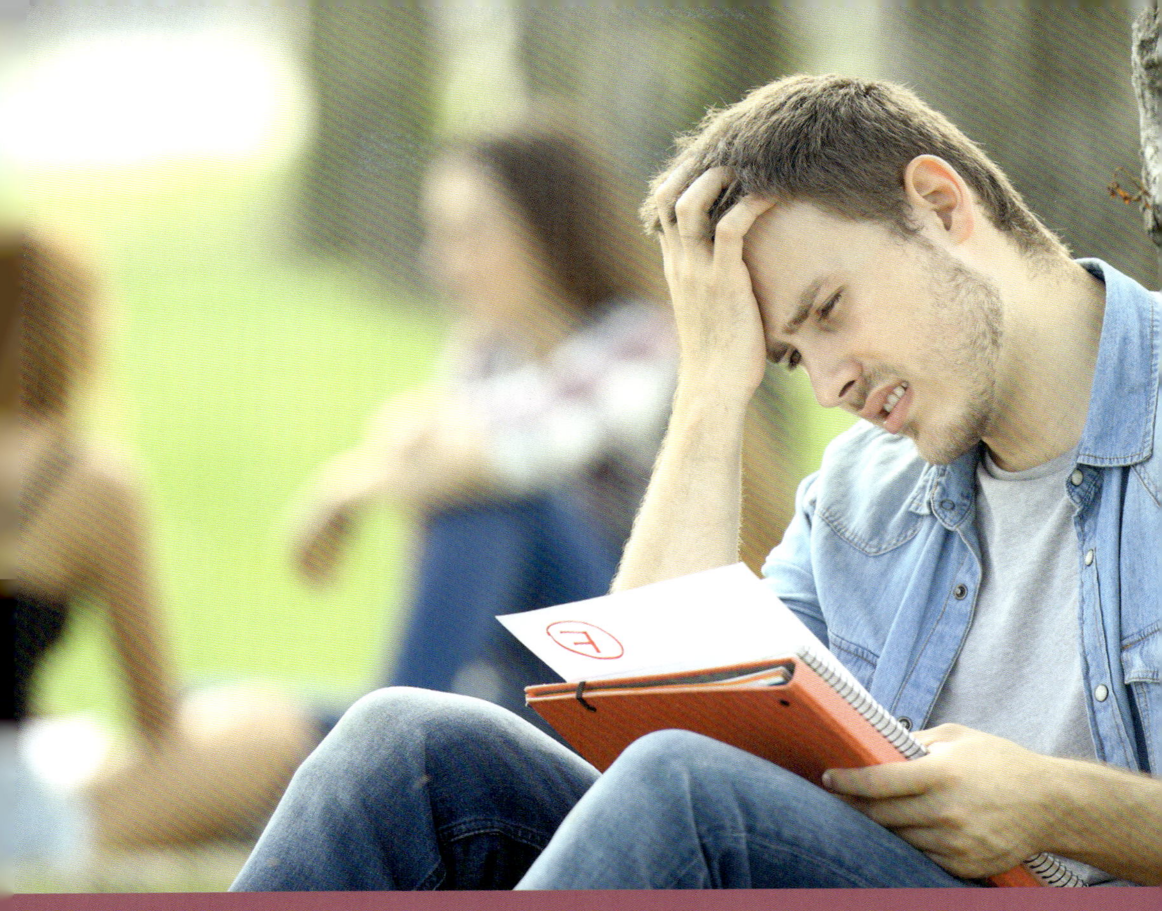

*Psychotic disorders can lead to challenges
at school.*

with psychotic disorders to feel ashamed

of their symptoms. They may pull away

from others. Stigma can make it difficult

to ask for help. It may prevent people

from seeking treatment. They may not tell

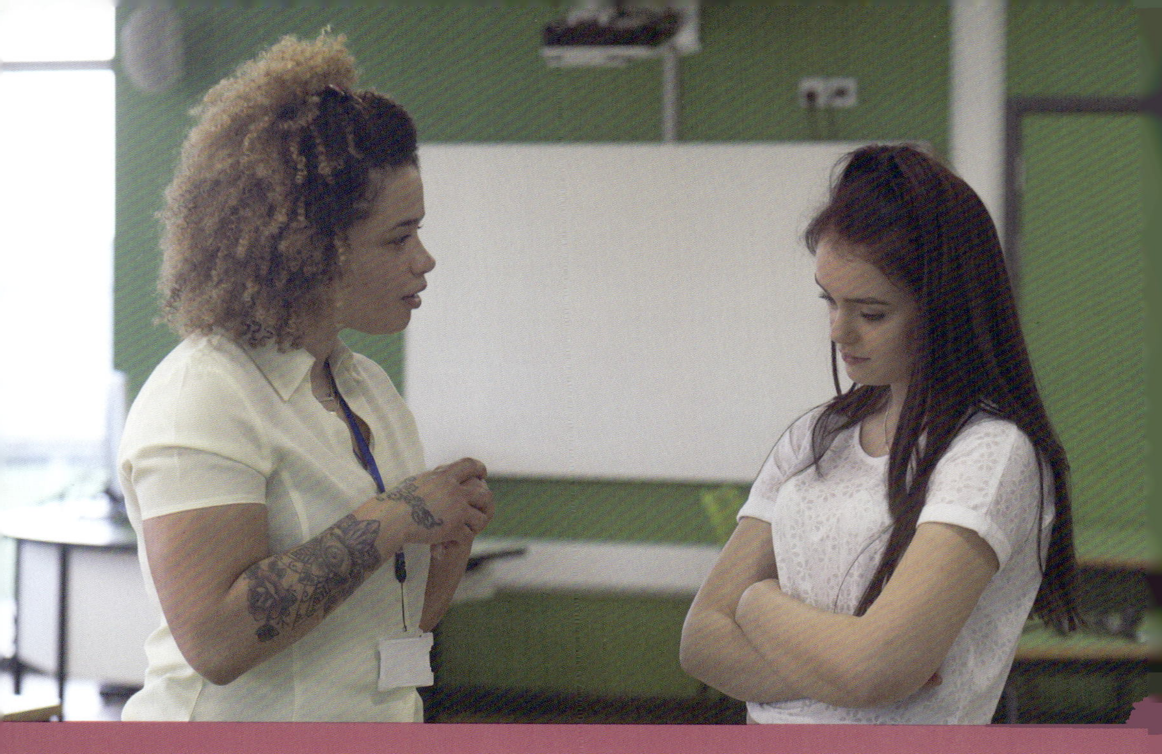

Teachers can help students with a psychotic disorder by creating a safe and positive environment.

others about their diagnosis. This can make recovery harder.

SCHOOL AND WORK

People experiencing psychosis may hear voices. These voices may interrupt thinking. They can make it difficult to concentrate.

Psychosis can affect memory. It can cause struggles at school. People may have trouble organizing their thoughts. Cecilia McGough talked about how schizophrenia affected her schoolwork. "Sometimes I wouldn't even be able to see the paper in front of my face because I was hallucinating too much," she said.[7]

Teachers may notice early stages of psychosis in their students. One sign is a sudden drop in grades. Students experiencing psychosis may say things that do not make sense. They may begin to have strange beliefs. Teachers should speak up if they notice these behaviors.

They should talk to the students' parents.

A psychotic disorder can also make it difficult to work. Schizophrenia is one of the leading causes of disability. Less than 15 percent of US adults with schizophrenia have a job. Many adults with schizophrenia want to work. But they struggle to find jobs. They may face stigma in the workplace. Sita Diehl works for the National Alliance on Mental Illness. She said, "The truth is that the majority of people with schizophrenia are willing and able to thrive in the workplace." [8]

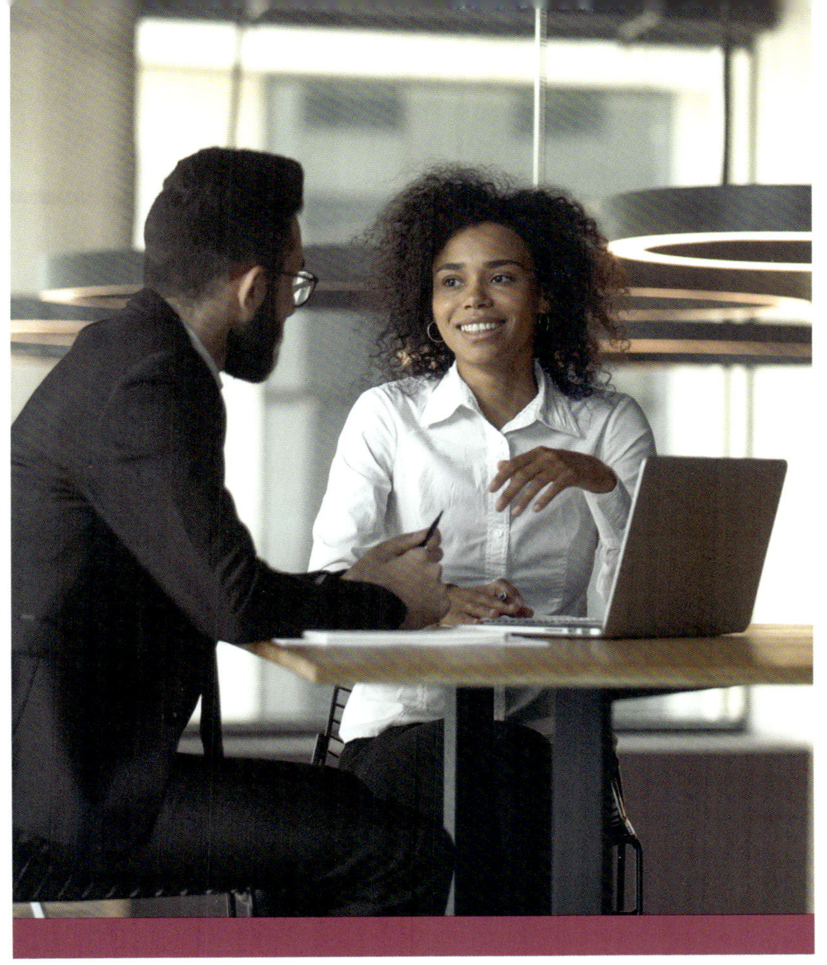

Employees should communicate with their employers about what they need in order to be successful.

Schizophrenia affects each person

differently. People need different

accommodations. Employers may offer

flexible work schedules. They can listen

to the needs of someone with a psychotic disorder. Together they can create a good working environment.

NAVIGATING RELATIONSHIPS

Psychosis can cause challenges in relationships. It can impact a person's mood. It can lower self-esteem. Someone experiencing psychosis may not want to socialize. Delusions may also cause him to be distrustful.

Other people may not understand psychosis. They may have negative beliefs about psychotic disorders. They may think that people with psychotic disorders are

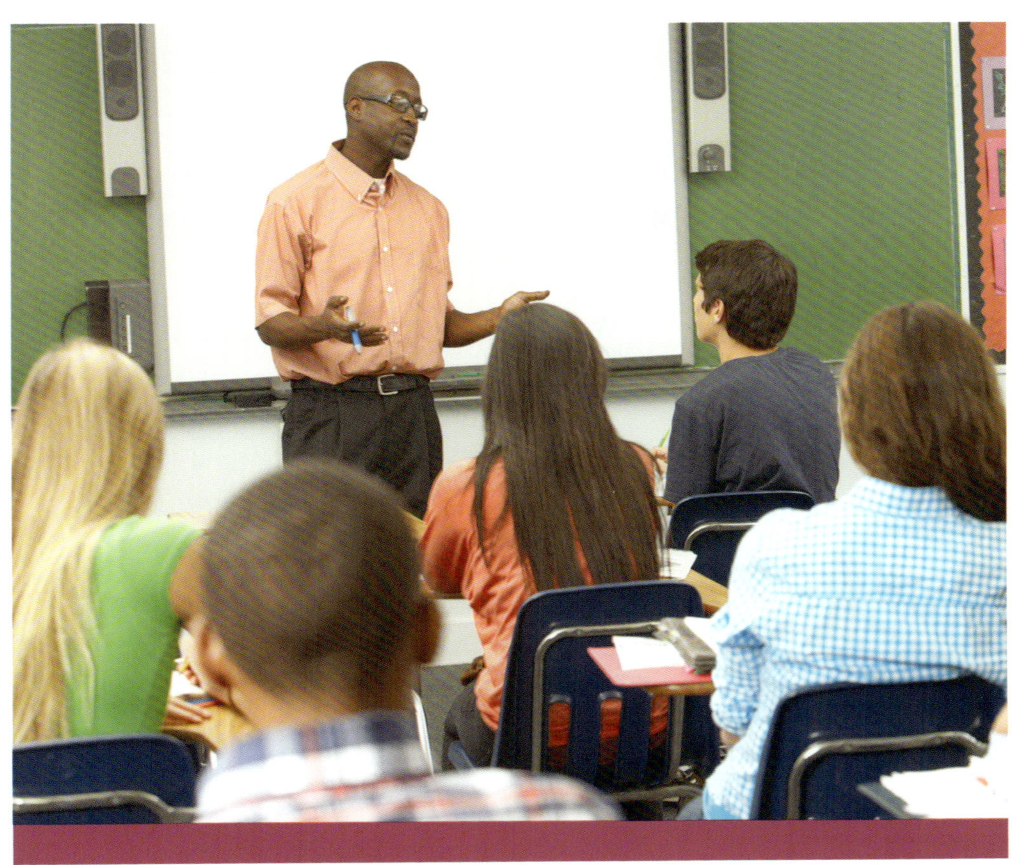

Increasing public education on psychotic disorders can help combat harmful stereotypes.

violent. They may not feel safe around them. But these **stereotypes** are untrue. They can hurt relationships. They can cause people with psychotic disorders to feel isolated.

Lack of support can increase the risk of suicide. Suicide is one of the leading causes of death in people with psychotic disorders. Treatment helps people cope with suicidal urges.

MENTAL ILLNESS AND THE MEDIA

Media may add to negative stereotypes about psychotic disorders. For example, the killer in a horror movie may have schizophrenia. This can lead people to think that people with this disorder are dangerous. But this is not true. Violent behaviors are extremely rare in people with schizophrenia. People are working to change how mental health is portrayed in entertainment. They want mental health professionals to review media so that it is accurate.

People with psychotic disorders may choose to share their diagnosis with others. Having a plan can be helpful. They figure out ways to explain their symptoms. These conversations can be difficult. But they can help others be more understanding.

Dr. David Crepaz-Keay was diagnosed with schizophrenia when he was a teen. He now works for the Mental Health Foundation. This organization works to end stigma surrounding mental health. He talked about ways to end stigma around psychotic disorders. "Moving the focus onto what people can do, rather than what they can't . . . is an important part of improving

our public image," he said.[9]

Social support can help someone handle

a psychotic disorder. Family and friends can

help a person cope. They may help him

avoid **triggers**. They listen when he talks

about his struggles. They encourage him to

get the help he needs.

SOCIETAL SUPPORT

Views on mental health have changed over

the years. The US government created

the Americans with Disabilities Act (ADA)

in 1990. This law protects people with

disabilities. This includes people with mental

illnesses. The ADA prevents employers from

firing an employee because of a diagnosis.

Employers must provide accommodations.

The ADA also requires equal access to

education and other services.

There are organizations that offer
support. They provide resources to people
with psychotic disorders. Schizophrenia
and Psychosis Action Alliance is one
organization. It shares information on
treatments. It increases public awareness.
This helps reduce stigma.

Living with a psychotic disorder can
be challenging. Laws and organizations
offer support. But people with psychotic
disorders can learn coping strategies.
They build support systems. They avoid
their triggers. They make healthy choices.
This includes avoiding drugs and alcohol.

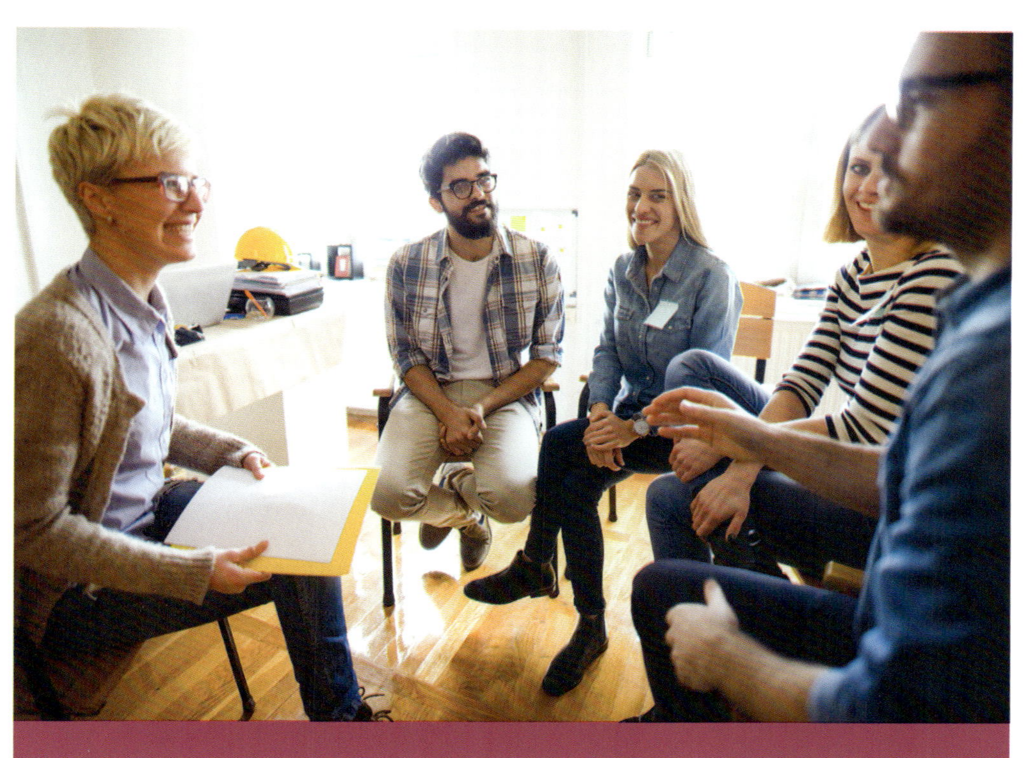

Sharing experiences with others can help people with psychotic disorders feel less alone.

They eat a balanced diet. They get a healthy amount of sleep. They work with a doctor to make a treatment plan. These steps help people with psychotic disorders have successful lives.

CHAPTER FOUR

TREATING PSYCHOTIC DISORDERS

The first step in treatment is to seek help. People experiencing psychosis can talk to a family member. They can go to a doctor. This step can be difficult. People experiencing psychosis may not understand that they need help.

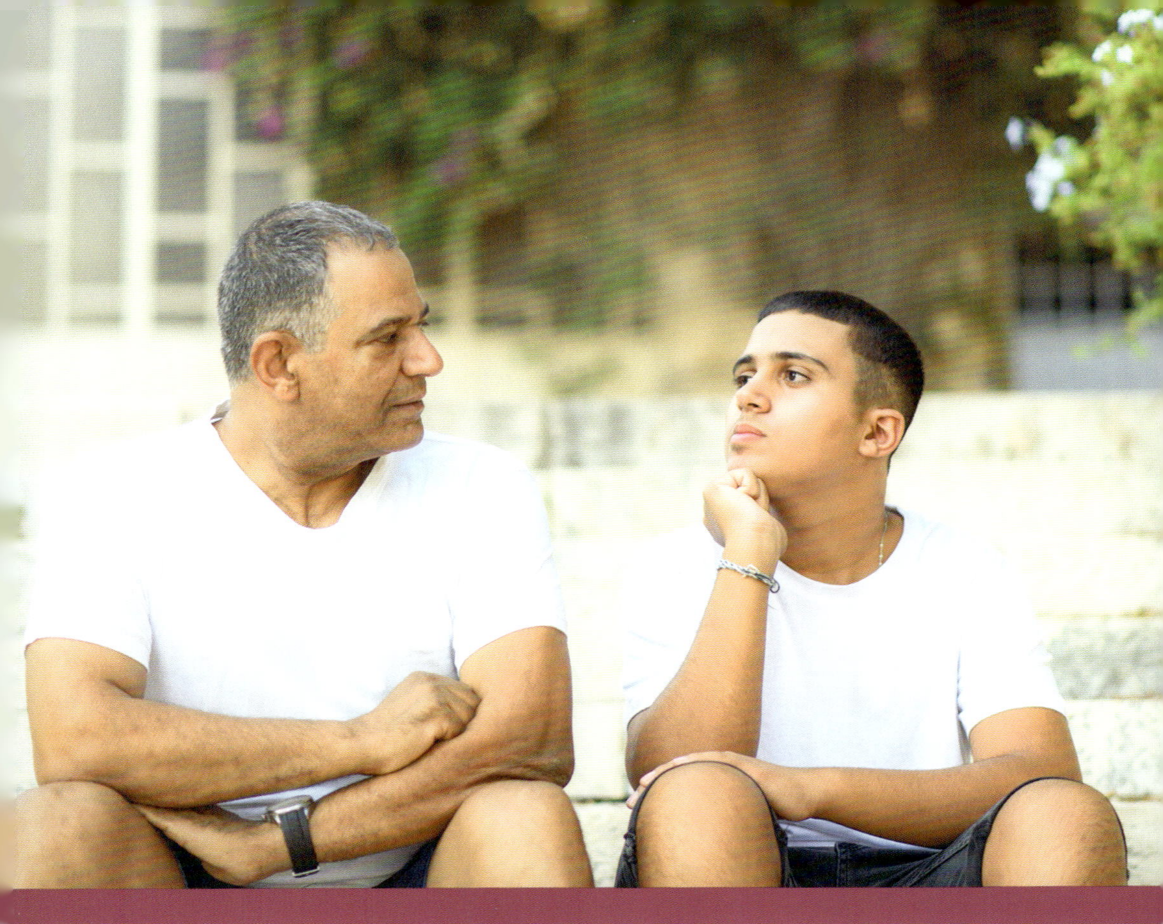

People who receive early treatment show the most improvement. This is why it is important to seek help. Mental health professionals help patients deal with their symptoms. They **prescribe** medications

and therapies.

MEDICATIONS

Treatment usually begins with medication. A

doctor prescribes antipsychotic drugs. One

type is CPZ. It blocks the brain chemical

INPATIENT CARE

People experiencing severe psychosis may
not be able to care for themselves. They may
need care in a hospital. This is called inpatient
care. They receive continuous care from mental
health professionals. Doctors can help patients
explore treatment options. Many patients
improve during their stays. Then they are able
to care for themselves.

dopamine. People with psychotic disorders usually have high levels of dopamine. New antipsychotic drugs also block dopamine. They help balance other brain chemicals.

Antipsychotic drugs can take effect quickly. They may lessen confusion within hours. It can take longer to get rid of other symptoms. Hallucinations and delusions take longer to treat. But many people stop having these symptoms after several weeks of taking medication.

Antipsychotics can cause side effects. People may experience drowsiness or dizziness. They may gain weight. Some

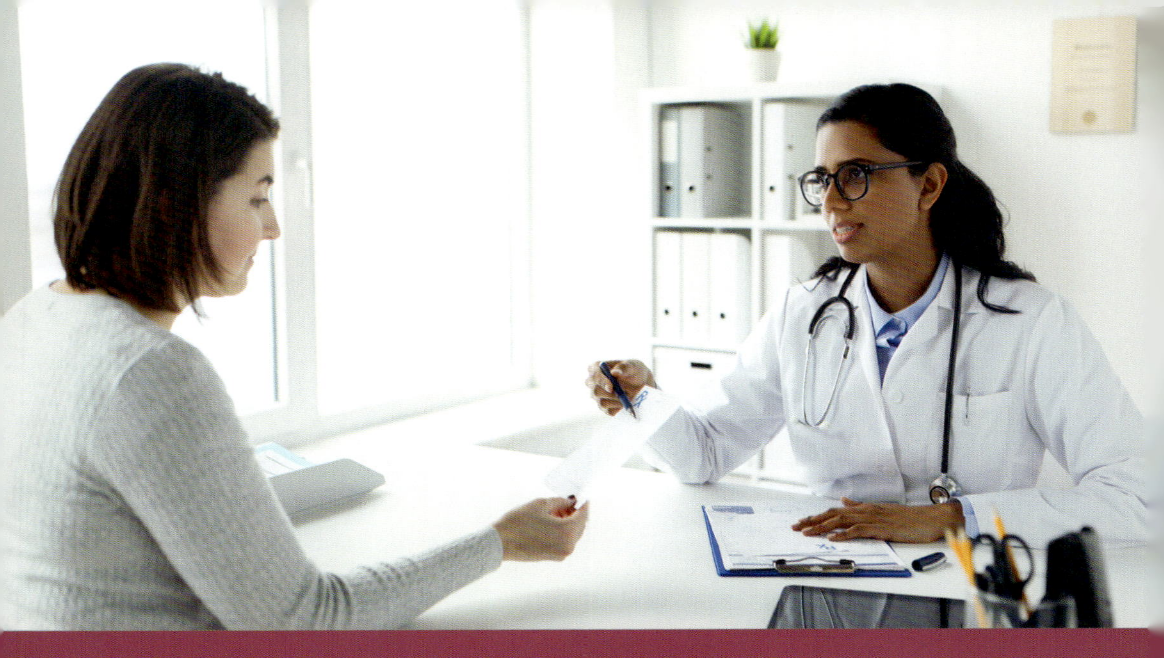

people begin to have problems with

movement. They may make jerky motions.

They may have trouble controlling facial

expressions. But new drugs have made

these effects rarer.

Negative symptoms are more difficult

to treat. Showing little emotion is one

example of a negative symptom. Another

is spending less time with others. Doctors may prescribe antidepressants to treat these symptoms.

Other medications also help with symptoms. Some people with psychotic disorders have anxiety. Doctors may prescribe anxiety medications. These drugs can also improve negative symptoms. Mood stabilizers are used to balance mood.

People with psychotic disorders may decide to stop taking medication. They may believe they are better. Or they may think the side effects are too severe. The decision to end medication should come

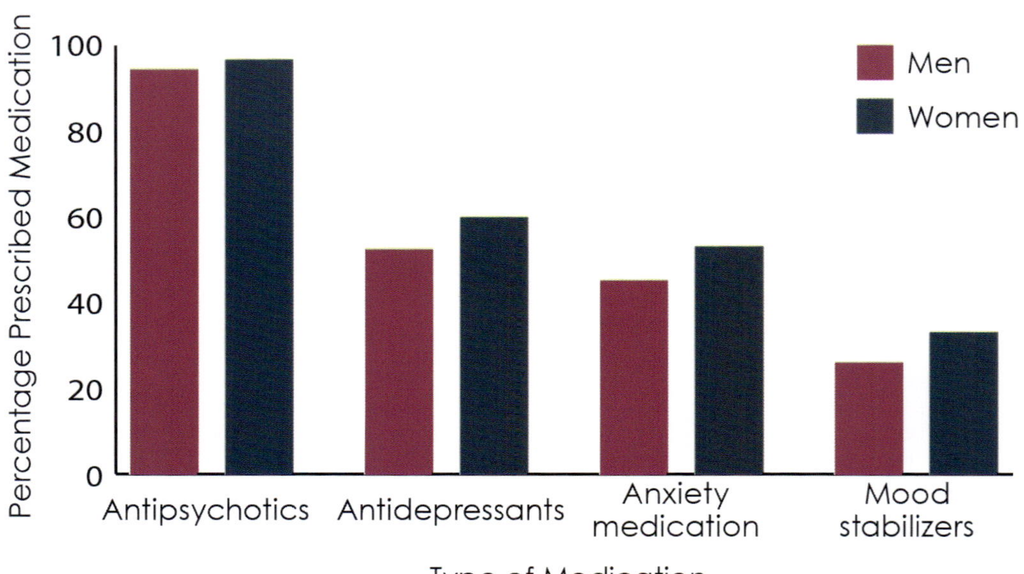

Source: Iris E. Sommer et al., "The Clinical Course of Schizophrenia in Women and Men—A Nation-Wide Cohort Study," NPJ Schizophrenia, May 1, 2020. www.nature.com.

A 2020 study looked at the medicines that men and women with schizophrenia used five years after their diagnosis. A person can take more than one form of medication.

from a doctor. Symptoms may return when

people stop taking medication. Doctors

and patients work together to find the best

medication. People respond to medicines and doses differently.

PSYCHOTHERAPY

Many people with psychotic disorders try psychotherapy. Talking to a therapist can help people cope with their symptoms. A combination of medication and therapy can be very effective. Cognitive behavioral therapy (CBT) is one type of therapy.

In CBT, patients learn to understand their thought processes. They begin to recognize their triggers. The patient and the therapist work together. They create goals. Patients may want to reduce feelings of shame. They

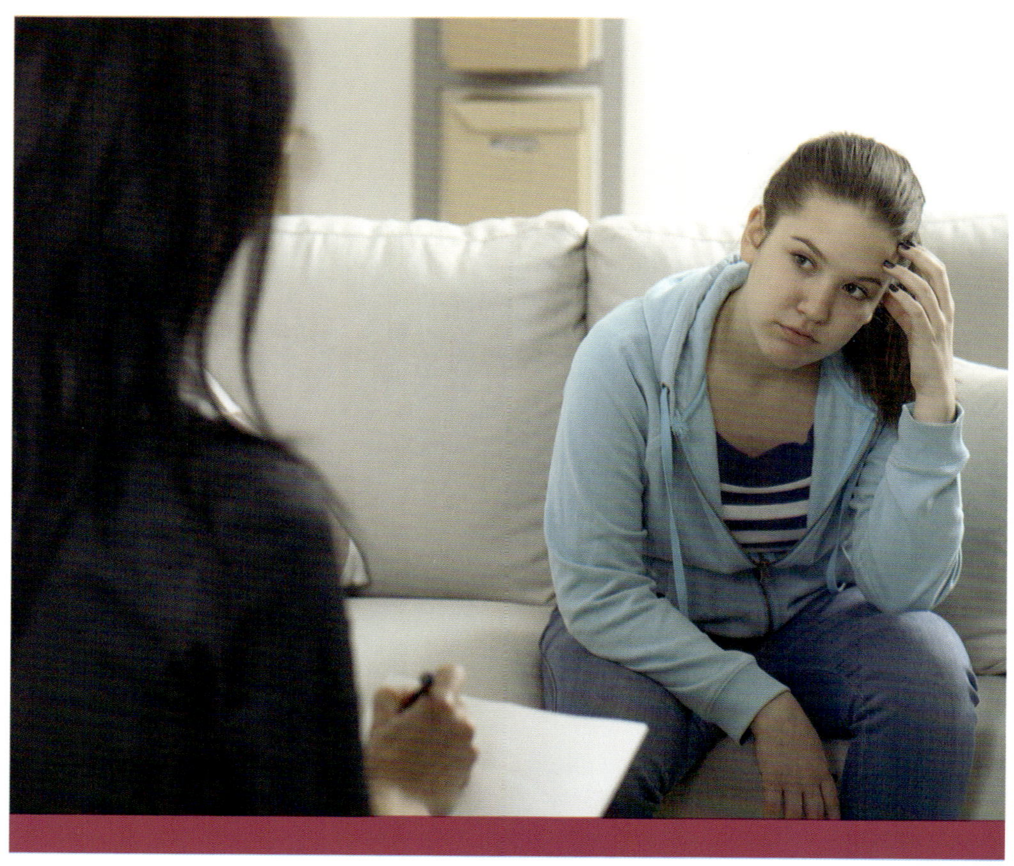

Therapy can help patients learn how to manage a psychotic disorder.

may want to return to work. The therapist

helps them meet these goals.

Family therapy can also be helpful. A

therapist meets with family members. They

learn how best to support their loved one.

They come up with ways to reduce stress.
Stress can worsen symptoms.

Some people with psychotic disorders try
group therapy. They meet with other people
who have psychotic disorders. They talk
about their struggles. They share coping
methods. A therapist oversees the group.
Group therapy can help deal with stigma.
Patients may feel less alone when hearing
about similar struggles.

OTHER TREATMENTS

Some patients with psychotic disorders do
not respond to medication. There are other
treatment options. Doctors may use ECT

to treat schizophrenia. They apply electric shocks to the brain. This can increase brain activity. It can reduce psychosis. Symptoms may improve within a week of treatment.

ECT can be expensive. It can also cause side effects such as memory loss. People may also have headaches after ECT. ECT is not used as a first treatment option for these reasons.

Transcranial magnetic stimulation can help treat hallucinations. Doctors place a magnetic coil on the patient's forehead. The coil produces electromagnetic pulses. This changes brain activity.

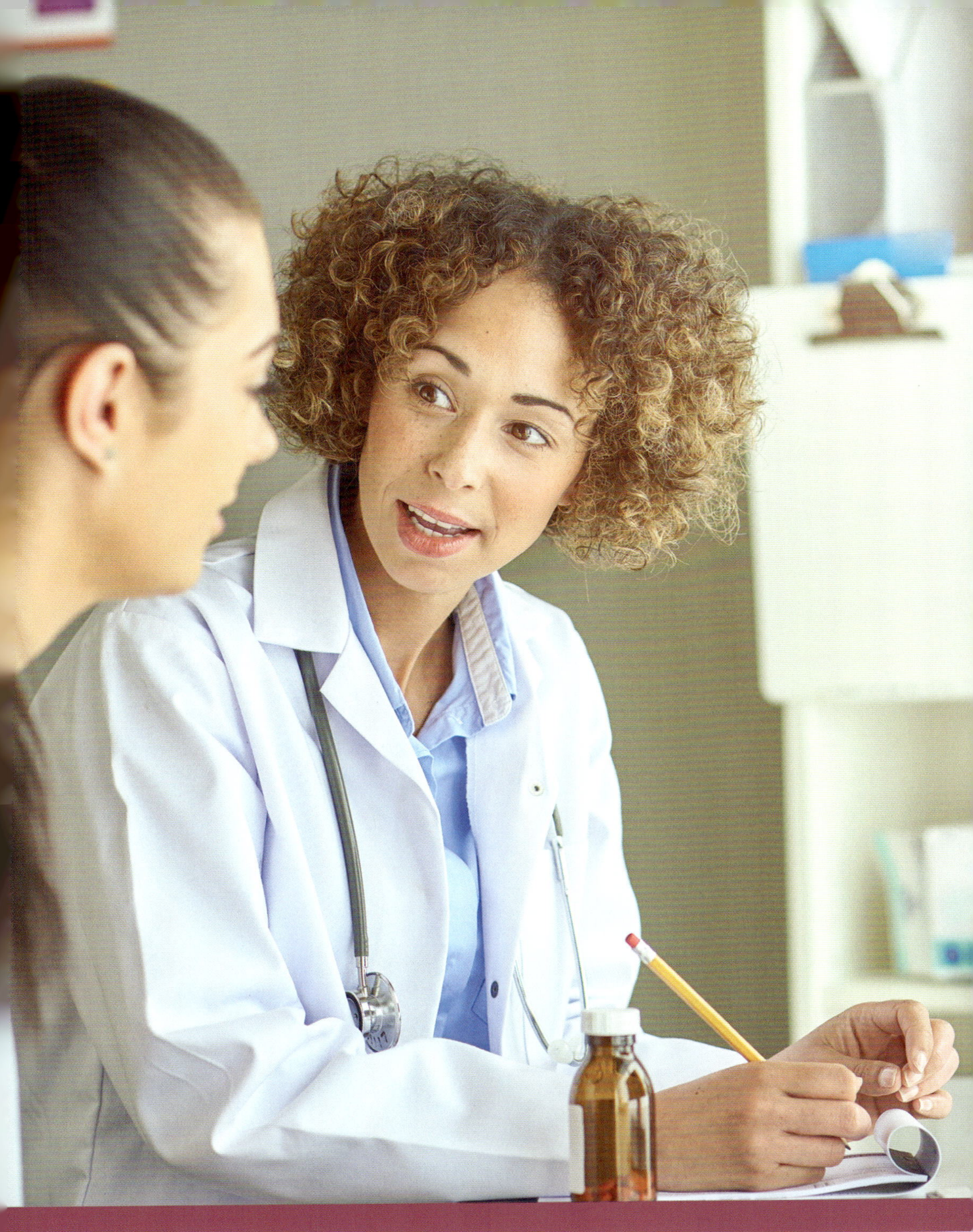

If medication is not effective, a doctor may suggest other forms of treatment.

ON THE HORIZON

Scientists continue to develop new treatments for psychotic disorders. Many antipsychotic drugs need to be taken daily. The drugs work for only a short time. Scientists hope to develop long-lasting antipsychotic drugs. These may be injected

VIRTUAL REALITY TREATMENTS

Some scientists believe that virtual reality (VR) can help with psychosis. Someone with a psychotic disorder can speak to a VR character. They can practice explaining their symptoms. They can work on social skills. They can use VR as a safe way to face their triggers. VR may be paired with other treatments in the future.

under the skin. They may be effective for

as long as three months. Long-lasting

drugs can make it easier to stick to a

treatment plan.

Negative symptoms are difficult to treat

with current medications. Research is

being done to create a drug to treat these

symptoms. The drug company Sunovion is

testing a new medicine. Scientists hope the

new drug can improve negative symptoms.

Scientists are also studying cognitive

remediation therapy (CRT). CRT may be

used to improve mental skills like attention.

It can help with memory. Computer

programs target the mental skills of patients.

The patients repeatedly train these skills.

This may help patients in real situations.

RECOVERY IS POSSIBLE

Many people with psychotic disorders learn
to manage their symptoms with treatment.
They learn to cope with stress. They take
steps to avoid triggers. Diet and exercise
can help reduce symptoms.

Michelle Hammer speaks about her
experience with schizophrenia. She wants
to end stigma surrounding psychotic
disorders. "It's been over eight years since

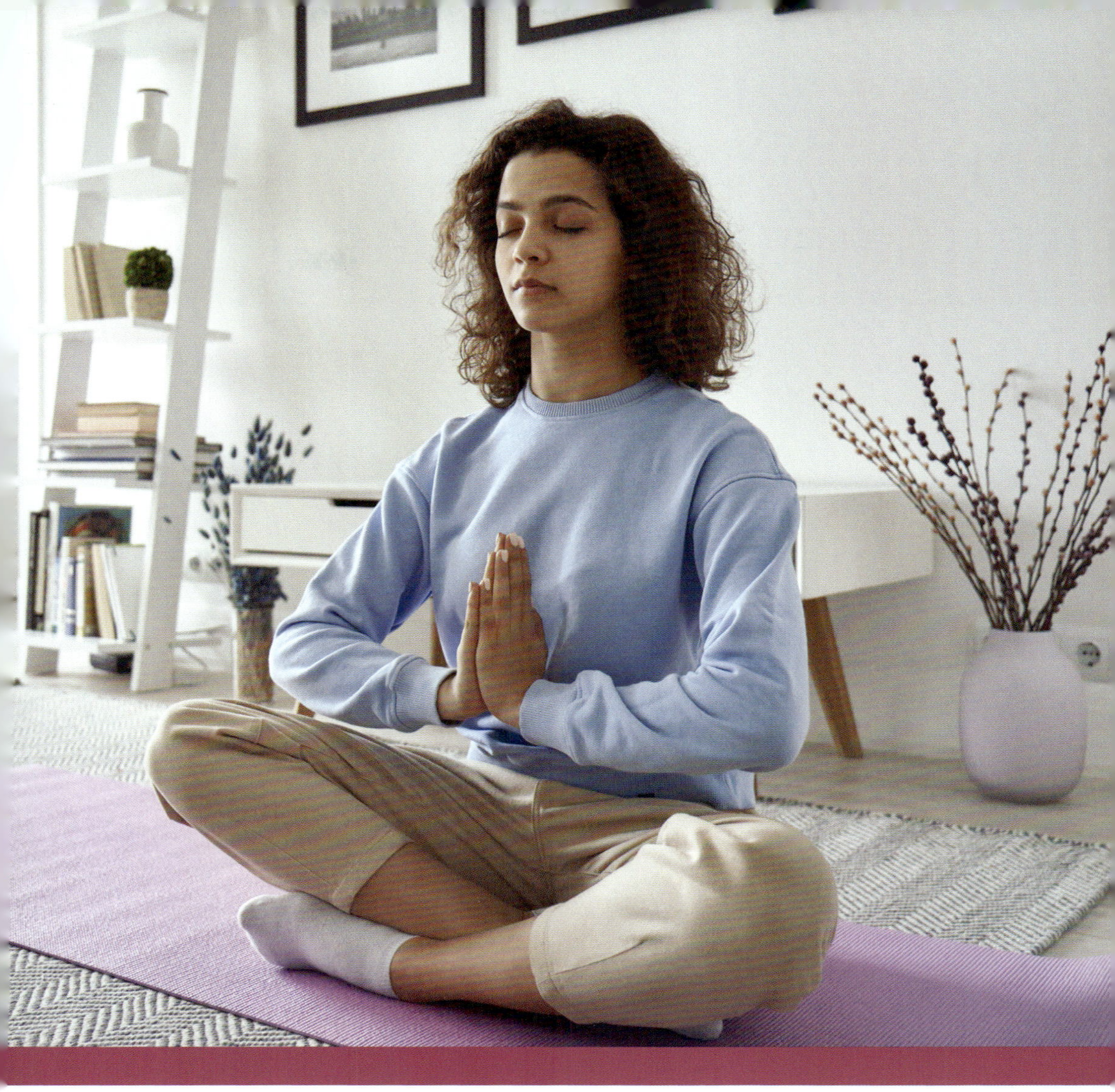

my schizophrenia diagnosis," Hammer said.

"I've learned to accept it and embrace it." [10]

GLOSSARY

asylums

institutions that historically cared for those with mental health disorders

diagnosed

identified a medical condition by examining symptoms

episode

a period of time during which someone is ill

hallucinations

images or sounds that are not real

prescribe

to instruct a patient to use a drug or other treatment

spectrum

a wide range

stereotypes

oversimplified beliefs about a group of people

stigma

a societal attitude about something that creates shame around it and makes people feel embarrassed to be associated with it

triggers

objects or situations that cause or bring about symptoms

SOURCE NOTES

INTRODUCTION: LIVING WITH SCHIZOPHRENIA

1. Quoted in TEDx Talks, "I Am Not a Monster: Schizophrenia," *YouTube*, March 27, 2017. www.youtube.com.

2. Quoted in TEDx Talks, "I Am Not a Monster."

3. Quoted in "Evil or Illness," *PBS*, 2021. www.pbs.org.

CHAPTER ONE: THE HISTORY OF PSYCHOTIC DISORDERS

4. Dorothea Dix, "'I Tell What I Have Seen,'" *American Journal of Public Health*, October 10, 2011. https://ajph.aphapublications.org.

5. Quoted in Warren Weaver Jr., "High Court Curbs Power to Confine the Mentally Ill," *New York Times*, June 27, 1975. www.nytimes.com.

CHAPTER TWO: NOTABLE PSYCHOTIC DISORDERS

6. Quoted in Brain & Behavior Research Foundation, "Schizophrenia: Potential Breakthroughs, Treatment, and Prevention," *YouTube*, February 27, 2018. www.youtube.com.

CHAPTER THREE: PSYCHOTIC DISORDERS AND EVERYDAY LIFE

7. Quoted in TEDx Talks, "I Am Not a Monster."

8. Quoted in Maria Hengeveld, "Job Hunting with Schizophrenia," *Atlantic*, July 28, 2015. www.theatlantic.com.

9. Quoted in Honor Whiteman, "Schizophrenia," *Medical News Today*, October 10, 2014. www.medicalnewstoday.com.

CHAPTER FOUR: TREATING PSYCHOTIC DISORDERS

10. Quoted in "Michelle Hammer's Essay Addresses Paranoid Schizophrenia," *This Is My Brave*, 2022. https://thisismybrave.org.

FOR FURTHER RESEARCH

BOOKS

Matt Chandler, *Understanding Mental Health*. Ann Arbor, MI: Cherry Lake
Publishing, 2020.

Kathy MacMillan, *Understanding Bipolar Disorder*. San Diego, CA:
BrightPoint Press, 2021.

Hilary W. Poole, *Schizophrenia*. New York: Weigl, 2018.

INTERNET SOURCES

"Schizophrenia in Children, Teens and Young Adults," *Healthy Children*,
July 28, 2021. www.healthychildren.org.

"Understanding Psychosis," *NIMH*, n.d. www.nimh.nih.gov.

"What's the Difference Between a Delusion and a Hallucination?" *Bright
Quest*, 2021. www.brightquest.com.

WEBSITES

Bring Change to Mind
https://bringchange2mind.org

This site contains educational resources for young people, including stories and tools on how to talk to others about mental illness.

National Alliance on Mental Illness
www.nami.org

This site provides descriptions of mental health conditions, including psychotic disorders. It also gives information on advocacy work.

Schizophrenia & Psychosis Action Alliance
https://sczaction.org

This site contains educational information and tools focused on the treatment and recovery of people experiencing psychosis.

INDEX

IMAGE CREDITS

Cover: © The Visuals You Need/
Shutterstock Images
5: © Motortion Films/
Shutterstock Images
7: © Fizkes/Shutterstock Images
9: © Olimpik/Shutterstock Images
10: © Fizkes/Shutterstock Images
13: © The Astonishing Ant-Man/
Shutterstock Images
15: © Trio Oean/iStockphoto
16: © Motortion Films/
Shutterstock Images
19: © Maridav/Shutterstock Images
21: © Clem Hencher-Stevens/
Shutterstock Images
24: © Nerthuz/Shutterstock Images
27: © Fizkes/Shutterstock Images
29: © SDI Productions/iStockphoto
31: © Narith 2527/iStockphoto
33: © Love Is/Shutterstock Images
35: © Diego Cervo/iStockphoto

37: © Damircudic/iStockphoto
38: © Raw Pixel/Shutterstock Images
40: © Aslysun/Shutterstock Images
45: © Antonio Guillem/
Shutterstock Images
46: © DGL images/
Shutterstock Images
49: © Fizkes/Shutterstock Images
51: © Monkey Business Images/
iStockphoto
57: © Dusan Petkovic/
Shutterstock Images
59: © Inna Reznik/Shutterstock Images
62: © Syda Productions/
Shutterstock Images
64: © Red Line Editorial
66: © Nikodash/Shutterstock Images
69: © Sturti/iStockphoto
73: © Insta Photos/
Shutterstock Images

ABOUT THE AUTHOR

Jennifer Phillips started out as a newspaper reporter in the Midwest. She now lives in Seattle, Washington, with her family. Phillips is an advocate for people with developmental disabilities and people with mental illness. She does her best writing in the early morning when the coffee is piping hot and the house is extremely quiet.